Alzheimer

Texte von / Texts by Fritz A. Henn, Christoph Ribbat und / and Sibylle Heeg

Peter Granser

A L Z H E I M E R

KEHRER

Dieser außergewöhnliche Bildband gewährt uns einen flüchtigen Blick auf die unterschiedlichen Gesichter der Alzheimer Demenz. Dieser Zustand, der für eine Mehrzahl von Heimeinweisungen verantwortlich ist, begegnet uns in vielen Erscheinungsformen. Krankheitsfälle mit einem klar definierten genetischen Ursprung beginnen in der Regel in jüngeren Jahren, oftmals bereits im fünften oder zu Beginn des sechsten Lebensjahrzehnts. Dies ist jedoch nur die Minderheit aller Fälle, während die Mehrzahl aller Erkrankungen keine genetische Ursache zeigen und erst mit vorangeschrittenem Alter Ende des sechsten Lebensjahrzehnts auftreten. Das Risiko, diese Krankheit zu entwickeln, steigt stetig bis zum 90sten Lebensjahr, wenn bereits mehr als 25% der Bevölkerung von diesem Leiden betroffen sind. Der sich entwickelnde Gedächtnisverlust und der Verlust des Orientierungsvermögens treffen uns im Kern unseres Selbstverständnisses. Die gezeigten Bilder dokumentieren den Mut und den Kampf dieser Patienten, und liefern Momentaufnahmen der erstaunlichen Würde, mit der sie dem Verlust ihrer Lebenserinnerungen gegenübertreten.

Peter Gransers Fotografien wollen den Verlust, den Alzheimerpatienten fühlen und erfahren müssen, nicht verbergen, sondern veranschaulichen den Schmerz, den Patienten und deren Angehörige erleiden. Gleichzeitig sind sie aber auch eine Anerkennung für die Bewahrung der menschlichen Würde unter denkbar schwierigsten Umständen. Sie helfen uns auch zu verstehen, welche Anstrengungen Familien bei der Pflege von Angehörigen, die von diesem Leiden betroffen sind, zu bewältigen haben. Letztlich ist es diese direkte Auseinandersetzung, die den Ansporn gibt, Forschungsanstrengungen nach Ursachen und Heilung voranzutreiben.

Jüngste Fortschritte in unserem Verständnis dieses Krankheitsbildes haben dazu beigetragen, therapeutische Ansätze zu liefern, die in der Lage sind, die Entwicklung der Erkrankung zu verlangsamen. Neue Erkenntnisse zur Entwicklung der Krankheit deuten darauf hin, dass wir Behandlungsmöglichkeiten auf der Spur sind, die das Fortschreiten der Erkrankung wirksam verhindern. Außerdem bringen uns heute mögliche detaillierte Studien auf molekularer und struktureller Ebene näher an unser Ziel heran, erkennen zu können, wer die Störung entwickeln wird, noch ehe sich erste signifikante Symptome zeigen. Dies wiederum eröffnet den Weg für präventive Behandlungsansätze, dem erklärten Ziel der Medizin. Indem wir uns mit diesem Problem auseinandersetzen und möglichen Lösungen stetig näher kommen, gelingt es uns hoffentlich auch, all denen Hoffnung zu bringen, die sich in den Fängen dieser Krankheit befinden – Patienten und ihren Familien.

Prof. Dr. Dr. Fritz A. Henn
Direktor des Zentralinstituts für Seelische Gesundheit, Mannheim, und
Sprecher des Kompetenznetzes Demenzen

In this book we glimpse at the varied faces of Alzheimer's Disease. This condition, which accounts for a majority of nursing home cases, has many forms. Cases with a clear genetic cause begin earlier in life often in the 50's and 60's. These are a small minority of the cases, while the majority of cases have no defined genetic cause and begin later in life toward the end of the sixth decade. The risk of developing this disease climbs through the nineth decade of life and at that point affects over 25% of the population. The developing memory loss and loss of orientation strike at our very sense of self. These pictures document the courage and struggle patients with the disorder face and record the remarkable dignity with which they face the loss of memories of their lives.

Peter Granser's photographies don't disguise the loss the patients feel and show the pain that they and their families suffer. At the same time they are a tribute to the preservation of human dignity in the most difficult of circumstances. They also help us understand the struggle families have in caring for loved ones afflicted with this condition. Facing this condition head on provides incentive to accelerate the research into its cause and cure.

Recent advances in our understanding have begun to provide therapies that slow the development of the disease. New knowledge about how the illness develops point in a direction that may lead to a treatment which effectively stops the progression of this disease. The detailed molecular and structural studies now possible are bringing us closer to the point of being able to predict who will develop the disorder prior to the onset of significant symptoms. This opens the possibility of preventive therapies, a goal toward which medicine continues to strive.

As we face the problem and begin to approach the solution we also bring hope to those caught in the throes of this disease; both patients and their families.

Prof. Dr. Dr. Fritz A. Henn

Director of the Central Institute of Mental Health, Mannheim, Germany and Speaker of the Competence Network Dementia, Germany

WO ICH DIE NACHT SCHLIEF   Peter Gransers Bilder von Alzheimer

1. „Was für ein lausiger Film", sagt der Mann zu seiner Frau und erhebt sich von seinem Platz. „Lass uns gehen." Seine Gattin aber antwortet, dass das unmöglich ist, macht keine Anstalten aufzustehen – und hat Recht. Das Paar sitzt nicht im Kino, sondern im Flugzeug. Sie sind auf dem Weg von New York City nach Amsterdam, unter ihnen erstreckt sich der Atlantik, der Film ist In-Flight-Entertainment, man kann nicht einfach gehen. Und dass der Mann trotzdem den Weg nach draußen sucht, ist kein Scherz, sondern bitterer Ernst und eine fast alltägliche Situation im Leben des alzheimerkranken Willem De Kooning und seiner Frau Elaine.

Das war 1983. De Kooning, geboren in Holland und als junger Mann in die USA emigriert, war einer der bekanntesten amerikanischen Maler seiner Zeit. Er hatte in den 1950er-Jahren seine ersten Erfolge gefeiert, war später jahrzehntelang schwerster Alkoholiker gewesen. Er trennte sich von Elaine, kam wieder mit ihr zusammen, trennte sich vom Alkohol, blieb bei Elaine, wurde dann mit Verdacht auf Alzheimer diagnostiziert. „Dein Körper wird stark bleiben", prophezeite ihm seine Frau unmittelbar nach dem Befund, „aber dein Gehirn wird sich langsam verabschieden." Mit beiden Vorhersagen lag sie richtig. Denn obwohl sich De Kooning immer weniger auf seine Erinnerungen und seine geistigen Fähigkeiten verlassen konnte, malte er weiter. Seine Augen, seine Muskeln schienen unabhängig von seinem Gehirn zu funktionieren. Er produzierte 341 Gemälde in einem Zeitraum von zehn Jahren – Bilder von fließenden Formen auf weißem Untergrund, in kräftigen, elementaren Farben. Sie sind leichter, optimistischer und fröhlicher als viele, die er in seinem Leben vor Alzheimer mit relativer Monotonie gemalt hatte. De Koonings Assistenten halfen ihm zwar in dieser Phase, stellten Materialien bereit, besserten Details nach. Aber der Schwung des Pinsels, die entscheidende Formgebung – sie kamen, trotz Alzheimer, von ihm. Die Distanz zu seinen Erinnerungen wurde größer und größer. In seinen Bildern aber war der Maler daheim.

2. Knapp zwei Jahrzehnte später, im Herbst des Jahres 2001, flog auch Peter Granser in die Niederlande. Wie elf weitere Kolleginnen und Kollegen aus allen Teilen der Welt war der junge Fotograf aus Stuttgart ausgewählt worden, an der „World Press Photo Masterclass" teilzunehmen, einem renommierten internationalen Workshop. In Gransers Gepäck auf der Reise nach Rotterdam: seine Bilder aus dem Stuttgarter Gradmann Haus, einer Wohneinrichtung für Alzheimerpatienten.

Von De Koonings Spätwerk hatte Granser nichts gewusst, als er daran ging, das alltägliche Leben seiner Protagonisten zu dokumentieren. Es ist Zufall, dass seine Fotografien in ihrer Klarheit und strahlenden Helligkeit den Gemälden des Amerikaners ähneln. Wie in jedem Jahr hatte die „Masterclass" ein Thema ausgegeben, das die jungen Fotografen zu behandeln hatten. 2001 war es recht modisch und hieß „Identität". Statt sich aber etwa mit dem Finden der Identität zu befassen – dem ersten Kuss, der ersten Hose von The Gap, dem ersten Semester – interessierte sich Granser für das weniger attraktive Ende des Spektrums: für Alzheimer, den Angriff auf die Identität also, den schleichenden, unaufhaltsamen Verlust des Selbst. Erst wollte er eine Alzheimer-Wohngemeinschaft in Berlin fotografieren. Dann, um vor Ort zu sein, entschied er sich für eine Serie über das Gradmann Haus ganz in seiner Nähe.

Warum das unhandliche Thema? Die Gründe haben viel mit Gransers Neugier zu tun. Anders als viele Dokumentarfotografen im deutschsprachigen Raum hat Granser nie eine Hochschule besucht. Er ist Autodidakt. Als 20-jähriger begann er, für die Lokalpresse zu arbeiten, fotografierte dann für überregionale Zeitungen, später für Magazine. Nebenher feilte er an freien Projekten, die nicht am Nachrichtenalltag entlang entwickelt wurden, aber eben auch nicht im Windschatten eines akademischen Lehrmeisters. Schnell gelang es ihm, eine eigene Handschrift zu entwickeln, mit schlichten, klaren Bildkompositionen, mit feiner Ironie. Granser interessiert sich für skurrile, künstliche Welten: das Touristenparadies Österreich, den New Yorker Vergnügungspark Coney Island, die Treffen von Deutschen, die sich am Wochenende als Cowboys verkleiden, um den Wilden Westen nachzuspielen.

Alzheimer war ein Sujet, auf das der Fotograf nicht ganz unvorbereitet war. Bevor er sich der Krankheit widmete, hatte er *Sun City* abgeschlossen, eine Serie über eine Rentnerkolonie im Südwesten der Vereinigten Staaten. In dieser seltsamen Stadt der fröhlichen Senioren war er zahllosen skurrilen Details begegnet. Und hatte dann Falten, Kakteen, Trockenhauben und Plastikflamingos zu einer ziemlich wahren und nur ein wenig übertriebenen Geschichte über die Zukunft des Alterns zusammengefasst. In *Sun City* heißt Senior-Sein nicht Innehalten, Zurückschauen, Abschied nehmen. Ganz im Gegenteil: in Gransers Bilderzählung tauchen lauter Damen und Herren auf, die sich ohne Kompromisse und ohne Larmoyanz radikal neu erfunden haben. Seine Arbeiten über Alzheimer loten das andere Extrem aus: die Abhängigkeit und die Verletzbarkeit. Wie in *Sun City* aber nähert sich Granser dieser Welt mit Staunen und nicht mit Zynismus.

3. Es gibt nicht viele Bildserien über Alzheimer. Und der Grund scheint offensichtlich. Zuallererst geht es bei dieser Krankheit um Sprache. Das ist es, was am meisten Angst macht: Alzheimer attackiert die kognitiven und intellektuellen Fähigkeiten und damit zuerst das Kommunikationsvermögen. Plötzlich gibt es Worte, die Erkrankte nicht mehr finden, schreiben, oder aussprechen können; plötzlich fallen ihnen Namen nicht mehr ein, sind schlicht verloren, wie von der Festplatte gelöscht. Um Sprache geht es auch bei der medizinischen Diagnose: um die einfachen Fragen, die der Arzt stellt, wenn er das sogenannte SIDAM-Interview zur Erkennung von Demenzerkrankungen durchführt („Welches Jahr haben wir?“ etwa, oder: „Wie hieß der erste deutsche Bundeskanzler der Nachkriegszeit?“). Falsche Antworten gelten dann schon als Symptome einer unheilbaren Krankheit, die die weitere Lebenserwartung im Mittel auf etwa acht Jahre verkürzt. Der Moment, in dem die Sprache versagt, markiert also den Beginn der unausweichlichen Tragödie, die durch Medikamente nur zeitweise aufgehalten werden kann. Deshalb ist da die Hilflosigkeit und das Erschrecken der Angehörigen, wenn alltägliche Gespräche plötzlich nicht mehr funktionieren. Der vertraute Mensch sieht genauso aus wie früher. Doch er redet wie ein Fremder.

Alzheimer kann jeden treffen und jeden, auch den wachsten Geist, verwirren. Das erklärt auch, warum in den letzten Jahren eine Flut von literarischen Texten über die Krankheit erschienen ist. Weil ihr Handwerkszeug die Sprache ist, fühlen sich Schriftsteller dem Thema offensichtlich besonders nah. Der Schweizer Martin Suter hat es in *Small World* zur Basis eines fesselnden Romans gemacht. Der amerikanische Autor Jonathan Franzen reagierte mit einem tief empfundenen Essay (*Das Gehirn meines Vaters*) und mit dem tragikomischen Bestseller *Die Korrekturen* auf die Demenz und den Tod seines Vaters. In einer aktuellen Kurzgeschichte der Kanadierin Alice Munro (*Der Bär kletterte über den Berg*) ist der erste Effekt von Alzheimer harmlos und komödiantisch – eine Frau macht sich kleine gelbe Post-Its an die Küchenschubladen: Hier ist das Besteck, hier sind die Geschirrtücher. Doch der Abschied von dieser Welt, das erzählt Munro in fast kühlem Ton, ist unaufhaltsam. Auch in ihrer Geschichte ist es das Versagen der Worte, das ihn besonders schmerzhaft macht.

4. Weil das Wort so viel gilt und das Bild so wenig, hatte Peter Granser mit diversen Vorbehalten zu kämpfen, als er im Gradmann Haus zu fotografieren begann. „Es gibt ein generelles Problem damit, wie Fotografen in der Öffentlichkeit gesehen werden“, sagt er. „Wer das Wort ‚Fotograf‘ hört, scheint zuerst zu denken: Der lauert Prominenten auf.“ Die Hausleitung konnte Granser relativ schnell von seiner vorsichtigen Arbeitsweise überzeugen – davon etwa, dass Scheinwerfer und Blitzlicht bei ihm keine Verwendung finden würden. Dann aber folgten die Gespräche mit den Angehörigen. „Die waren schwieriger“, erinnert er sich. „Was ist, wenn das jemand sieht?“, wurde der Fotograf gefragt. Familienmitglieder machten sich Sorgen über die Reaktionen von Freunden, Kollegen, Bekannten. Granser besuchte die Einrichtung Tag für Tag, zeigte die entstandenen Bilder, erklärte sein Konzept, bis sich die Angehörigen nach und nach von ihren Bedenken lösten. Ein Gespräch ist ihm besonders in Erinnerung geblieben: „Eine Frau sagte, wie sehr ihr eins meiner Bilder geholfen habe, den Kampf ihres Mannes mit Alzheimer zu akzeptieren. Vorher, sagte sie, habe sie immer krampfhaft an dem alten Bild festgehalten, das sie noch von ihm im Kopf hatte.“

Eines räumt der Fotograf ein: Der Schauplatz seiner Serie kann nicht unbedingt als repräsentativ gelten. Das Gradmann Haus ist ein Modellprojekt. Es beherbergt nur 24 permanente Bewohner und eine Tagesgruppe von 10 bis 15 Erkrankten. Die Architektur ist abgestimmt auf ihre Bedürfnisse: mit viel Tageslicht, einem Garten, mit langen Gängen, die dem Bewegungsdrang von Alzheimerpatienten entgegenkommen. Allein im Stuttgarter Raum gibt es Tausende von Betroffenen, für die eine solche Betreuung ein Segen wäre. „Es ist nicht typisch, aber es sollte typisch sein“, sagt Granser. „Ich wollte nicht die Pflegestationen zeigen, die die Kranken schlicht ans Bett schnallen. Mir ging es um einfachere Bilder, die aber doch einen Zugang vermitteln zu dieser Krankheit und zu der Abgeschlossenheit, in der die Leute leben.“

Um diesen Zugang zu eröffnen, hat Granser seine Serie sorgsam ausgewogen. Einerseits stellen die Bilder die menschliche Person und das, was sie aushalten muss, in den Vordergrund. Andererseits respektiert der Fotograf jederzeit die Würde des Patienten. Pastellige Farben umschmeicheln die Männer und Frauen; unaufdringlich begleitet der Blick ihren Gang, ihre Gesten. Die Frau, die mit ihrem Kot ihr Zimmer beschmiert, der Mann, der in den Krankenhausflur pinkelt, weil ihm das Konzept „zur Toilette gehen" nicht mehr präsent ist – diese Szenen erscheinen bei Granser nicht. Er wusste, was er nicht wollte: eine Fortführung der konventionellen Reportagefotografie der 1960er- und 1970er-Jahre, die mit fast befremdender Vorliebe das Elend, die Nacktheit und die Schwäche von Menschen dramatisiert „Gute Fotografie ist zwar immer voyeuristisch", sagt der Fotobuch-Verleger Chris Boot, der Gransers Projekt in der „World Press Photo Master Class" kennen lernte. „Peters Bilder aber sind weder aggressiv noch sentimental."

Farbe spielt bei diesem Balanceakt eine zentrale Rolle. Sie ist wie ein Schleier, der die Dargestellten schützt. Zudem hilft sie dem Fotografen, genau der klassischen Sozialreportage aus dem Weg zu gehen, die Bilder von Geisteskrankheit und Demenz stets mit Graustufen der Düsternis umgibt. „Irgendwann habe ich gemerkt", so Granser, „dass diese großen Vorbilder aus der Schwarzweißfotografie mir nicht bei den Geschichten helfen, die ich erzählen muss." Gransers helle Farben schaffen Distanz: „Sie heben die Bilder über die Realität", sagt der Fotograf. Kein Anspruch auf Allgemeingültigkeit wird erhoben. Dies ist nur ein Ansatz, eine Perspektive, eine Version von Alzheimer.

Die unhandliche Mittelformatkamera unterstützt diese behutsame Strategie noch einmal. Die Aufnahmen sind Dokumente langer Tage, entstanden bei manchmal komplett ereignislosen Besuchen, bei denen Peter Granser nur zwei-, dreimal auf den Auslöser drückte. Mit Kamera und Stativ bewegte er sich langsam durch die Flure, ließ sich von Bewohnern an die Hand nehmen und herumführen. Er betrachtete den Nachttisch einer Dame: das gerahmte Foto ihres Gatten, den „Danone Gran Frutta"-Joghurtbecher, die Einwegtaschentücher von Schlecker, den Kamm, den Lippenstift, das Blumengesteck. Er fotografierte Bewegungen aus der Distanz: das ziellose Suchen, die heraufzuckenden Hände. Und er vermied Hektik und Konfrontation.

5. Gransers Portraits allerdings sind von atemberaubender Unmittelbarkeit. Es ist fast unmöglich, sich nicht von diesen Gesichtern in den Bann schlagen zu lassen, sich nicht hineinzudenken in die Lebensgeschichten, für die sie stehen. Manche Beobachter werden Schwierigkeiten mit diesen Nahaufnahmen haben: Schließlich gibt es in der aktuellen Dokumentarfotografie eine Art ungeschriebenes Gesetz, dass die Beziehung zwischen Fotografierendem und Fotografierten stets gleichberechtigt sein soll. Das Portrait, daran hat man sich gewöhnt, hat diese Gleichberechtigung ausdzurücken. Und Portraitisten menschlicher Seltsamkeiten werden heute schnell als herablassend wahrgenommen, weil die Kamera schon zu oft dazu benutzt worden ist, Menschen zu entblößen, sie durch das Bild zu demütigen, sie aufgrund ihrer Rasse, ihrer sozialen Herkunft, ihres mentalen Zustands als minderwertig zu kategorisieren. Daher zeigen die Portraits der aktuellen Dokumentarfotografie meist extrem selbstbewusste Individuen, die das Objektiv mit solcher Energie und Furchtlosigkeit anstarren, bis es dem Betrachter fast bange wird.

Bei den Portraitsitzungen im Gradmann Haus ging es anders zu. Da wusste nur einer, was wirklich geschah: der Fotograf (nur zwei Bewohner hatten eine ungefähre Vorstellung davon, was dieser junge Mann eigentlich trieb, der da in den Fluren und Aufenthaltsräumen unterwegs war). Weil die Portraitierten ahnungslos sind, wird zum einen die Künstlichkeit des fotografischen Akts aufgehoben. Die Männer und Frauen präsentieren sich nicht, bieten ihr Gesicht nicht an, sind getrieben von der Ruhelosigkeit, die Alzheimer ihnen diktiert. Das mag authentische Portraits garantieren. Zum anderen aber könnten Kritiker sich in den Block notieren, dass es sich hier fast um eine Rückkehr zu den Bildern des späten 19. Jahrhunderts handelt, als Fotografen scharenweise ausschwärmten, um die Geisteskranken ihres Zeitalters per Bild zu katalogisieren.

Um dieses Argument ernsthaft zu verfolgen, müsste man Peter Gransers Bilder konsequent ignorieren. Es gibt nur wenige Portrait-Serien zeitgenössischer Fotografen, in denen den Protagonisten so viel Würde und so viel Autorität zugebilligt werden. Zwar weiß Granser im Moment der Aufnahme viel mehr als die von ihm Abgebildeten. Zwar kontrolliert er eine Situation, die sie nicht durchschauen. Aber was wäre die Alternative? Wenn Journalisten und Literaten über Alzheimerpatienten schreiben, dann operieren sie auf der Basis eines noch viel eklatanteren Missverhältnisses. Der Autor zieht alle Register seines sprachlichen Vermögens, drückt sich aus, bringt auf den Punkt – der Patient erscheint dagegen schon deshalb als fehlerhaftes Wesen, weil er ausgeschert ist aus der Welt der Sprache. Auguste D. ist es so gegangen, der Patientin von Alois Alzheimer: Mit ihren falschen Antworten auf einfache Fragen („Wie heißt Ihr Mann?" – „Ich glaube, Auguste.") beginnt die Geschichte dieser Krankheit im Jahr 1901. Mit der Schriftstellerin Iris Murdoch geschah Vergleichbares: Als Murdochs Gatte John Bayley in seinem viel gelesenen autobiografischen Werk *Elegie für Iris* von ihr berichtete, hatte er das letzte Wort, weil ihm ihre Krankheit erspart geblieben war. Und die Welt lernte Murdoch, die Philosophin und weltberühmte Autorin, als verwirrte alte Dame kennen, die apathisch auf dem Sofa sitzt und erst dann einen Ausdruck von Freude zeigt, wenn die tägliche Folge der „Teletubbies" beginnt. In Peter Gransers Bildern entsteht ein solches Ungleichgewicht nicht. Der Fotograf bleibt unsichtbar, die Protagonisten anonym.

6. Wir sind daran gewöhnt, uns Alzheimer als – noch – unheilbare Geißel der Menschheit vorzustellen. Unsere Hoffnungen setzen wir auf die ambitionierten Mediziner, die in Laboratorien weltweit an Diagnosemethoden arbeiten, die eine frühzeitige Therapie ermöglichen können. Und dann ist da noch das Fernziel: jenes Medikament, das die Krankheit einmal heilen können soll. Wir sind uns sicher: Eines Tages ist es so weit. Die Zukunft also mag farbig sein (lassen die Forscher verlauten); nur der Alzheimer-Alltag ist grau.

Es gibt aber auch andere Stimmen. Der Wissenschaftsjournalist David Shenk argumentiert, dass jenes hypothetische Anti-Alzheimer-Wundermittel der Menschheit gar nicht so viel helfen würde. Shenk fragt, ob die Phase des Vergessens nicht vielleicht so selbstverständlich zum Ende des Lebens gehört wie das Lernen zu seinem Beginn. Für ihn klingt der Plan, die Senilität zu besiegen, wie die Idee, den Winter abschaffen zu wollen. 419 vor Christus verkündete Aristophanes, dass alte Männer wieder zu Kindern werden. Zu Beginn des 17. Jahrhunderts ließ Shakespeare seinen alten König Lear wie einen Alzheimerpatienten mit dem Alltag hadern: „All mein Verstand“, klagt Lear, „entsinnt sich dieser Kleider nicht; noch weiß ich / Wo ich die Nacht schlief.“ Wenn die Auseinandersetzung mit der Demenz seit Jahrtausenden zu unserer Kultur gehört, wenn die Freuden des Lebens nur deshalb so groß sind, weil wir wissen, was am Ende auf uns zukommt: Warum dann das Verlangen danach, in diese Prozesse einzugreifen?

Vergessen, die Kehrseite des Erinnerns, macht unser Menschsein mit aus. Manche Beobachter halten den Kampf gegen Senilität deshalb nicht für die wichtigste Schlacht, die die Menschheit nun ausfechten muss. Wer die Krankheit mit AIDS vergleicht, wird vorsichtig sein, von Alzheimer als weltweiter Epidemie zu sprechen, die Millionen von Menschen dahinrafft. Anders als AIDS ist Alzheimer nur ein Konstrukt – ein künstliches Label, benutzt von Medizinern, die irgendwann beschlossen haben, Altersdemenz nicht mehr als naturgegeben hinzunehmen, sondern als Krankheit zu definieren und zu bekämpfen. Anders als AIDS im südlichen Afrika ist Alzheimer keine Katastrophe, die unsere Gesellschaft zugrunde zu richten droht, sondern eine soziale Herausforderung. So könnte man die Dinge relativieren.

Solche Anstöße motivieren manche Beobachter dazu, neu über Demenz nachzudenken: sie nicht nur als zu vernichtenden Feind zu sehen, sondern als Selbstverständlichkeit im menschlichen Leben. In den USA leitet die Altenforscherin Anne Davis Basting das Projekt „Time Slips“: Sie organisiert Gesprächsrunden von Alzheimerpatienten, in denen diese kollektiv Geschichten erzählen, die zerfasert sind, zusammenhanglos und improvisiert, aus denen dann aber Theaterstücke entstehen. Basting will so demonstrieren, wie starr und letztlich künstlich unsere Vorstellung davon ist, dass Individualität und Kreativität ganz und gar von einem perfekt funktionierenden Verstand abhängig sind. Das schließlich zeigen Willem De Koonings späte Gemälde: Es gibt eine Form von künstlerischem Ausdruck, die den klaren, rationalen Verstand nicht braucht. Auch Peter Gransers Bilder sind in diesem Zusammenhang zu verstehen – als eindrucksvolle Versuche, Demenz neu zu sehen, ohne Scheu und ohne Panik.

Für viele Angehörige von Alzheimerkranken dürften diese Gedanken arg seltsam klingen. Zwei von drei Demenzpatienten leben Zuhause, werden von Familienmitgliedern gepflegt. Wer einen Erkrankten nur einen Tag lang betreut hat, weiß um die düsteren, hässlichen Seiten der Krankheit. Das Vergessen als Teil des Lebens akzeptieren? Alzheimer als Konstrukt begreifen, gar als Chance für neue Kreativität? Das, könnte man einwenden, kann nur Theoretikern einfallen. Darauf kommt nur jemand, der noch nicht von der eigenen Mutter gefragt wurde, ob man sich schon einmal irgendwo gesehen habe. Denn der Prozess des Vergessens ist beileibe nicht nur friedlich und harmonisch. Immer mehr konzentriert sich auch die Forschung auf die zahlreichen schwerwiegenden Symptome, die den Erinnerungsverlust begleiten. Angstzustände entstehen, Depressionen, Verfolgungswahn – und Zorn und Gewaltbereitschaft, die sich gegen die Angehörigen richten, selbst wenn sie die Kranken mit der größten Hingabe pflegen. Davon, so könnte man sich beklagen, sieht man hier nichts.

Die Einwände machen Sinn in der generellen Debatte über Alzheimer. Sie gehen jedoch ins Leere, was Peter Gransers Serie betrifft. Denn diese verspricht kein umfassendes Panorama. Sie will auch keine wissenschaftliche Studie sein. Behutsam, nüchtern und optimistisch beginnt sie einen Dialog und richtet den Blick auf Gesichter und Gesten, die sonst niemand betrachten würde. Hochstapelei ist Gransers Sache nicht. Noch einmal: Dies ist nur eine Geschichte über die Spuren, die Alzheimer hinterlässt. Sie handelt von Verlorenheit. Sie handelt von Würde. Und von der strahlenden Widersprüchlichkeit des menschlichen Gesichts.

Christoph Ribbat
publiziert zu amerikanischer Erzählliteratur, Fotografie und Kulturgeschichte und lehrt an der Universität Bonn.

Für Hilfe und Hinweise dankt der Autor Peter Granser, Gabriele Kreutzner, Ina Schermuly, Jochen Klucken, Alberto Lleo und Chris Boot. Unverzichtbar war David Shenks herausragendes Buch *The Forgetting: Alzheimer's – Portrait of an Epidemic* (New York, 2001).

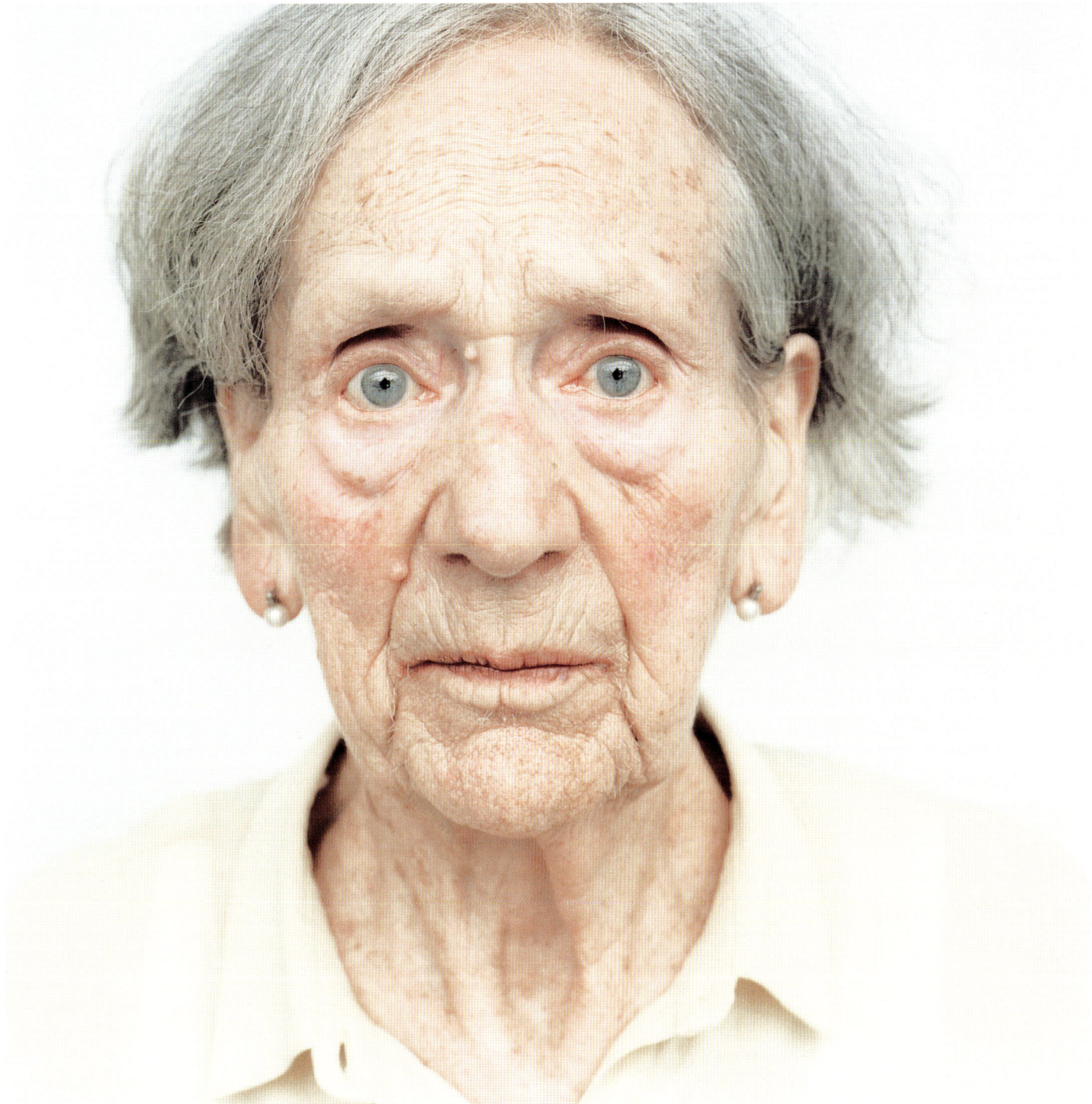

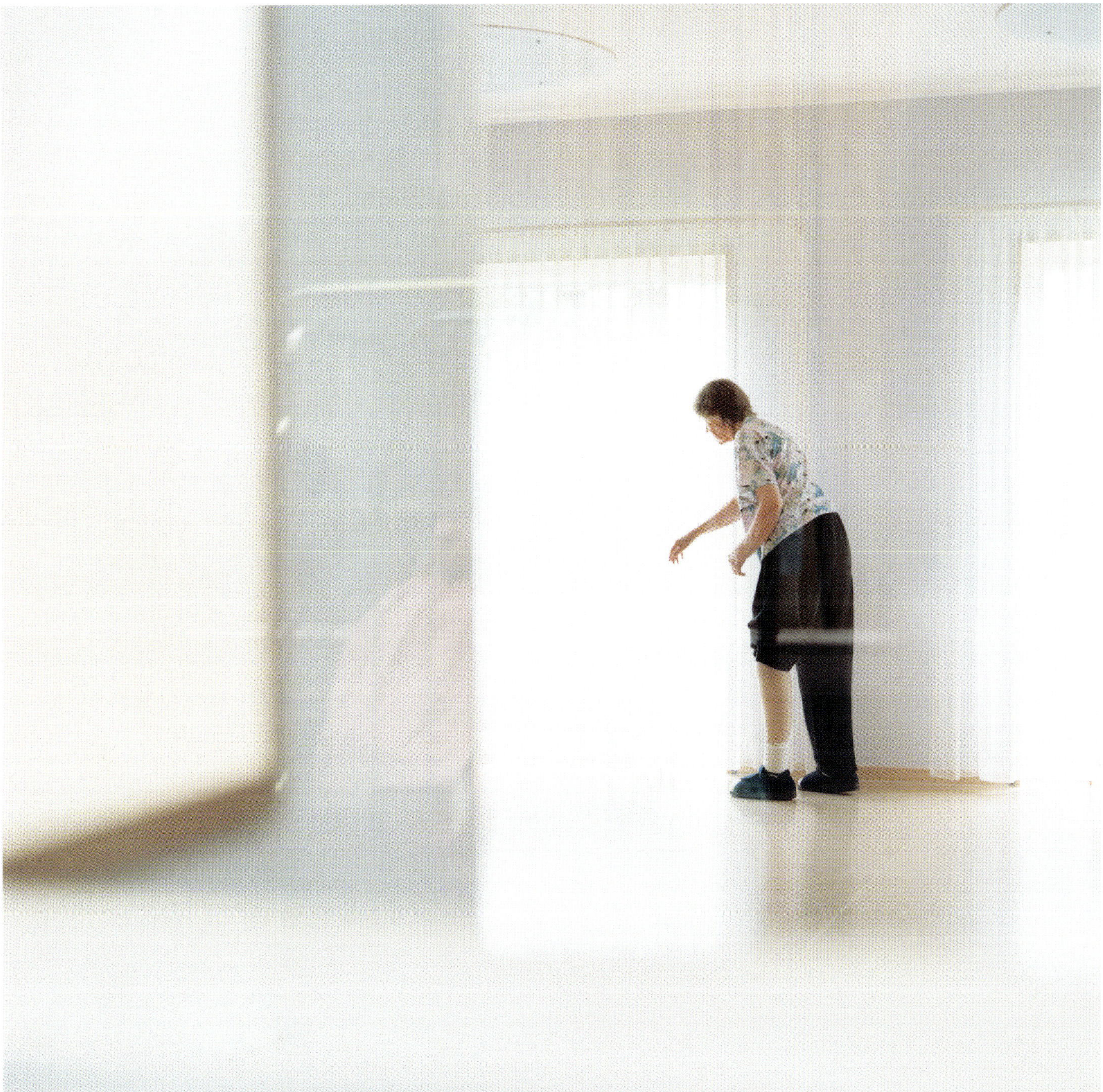

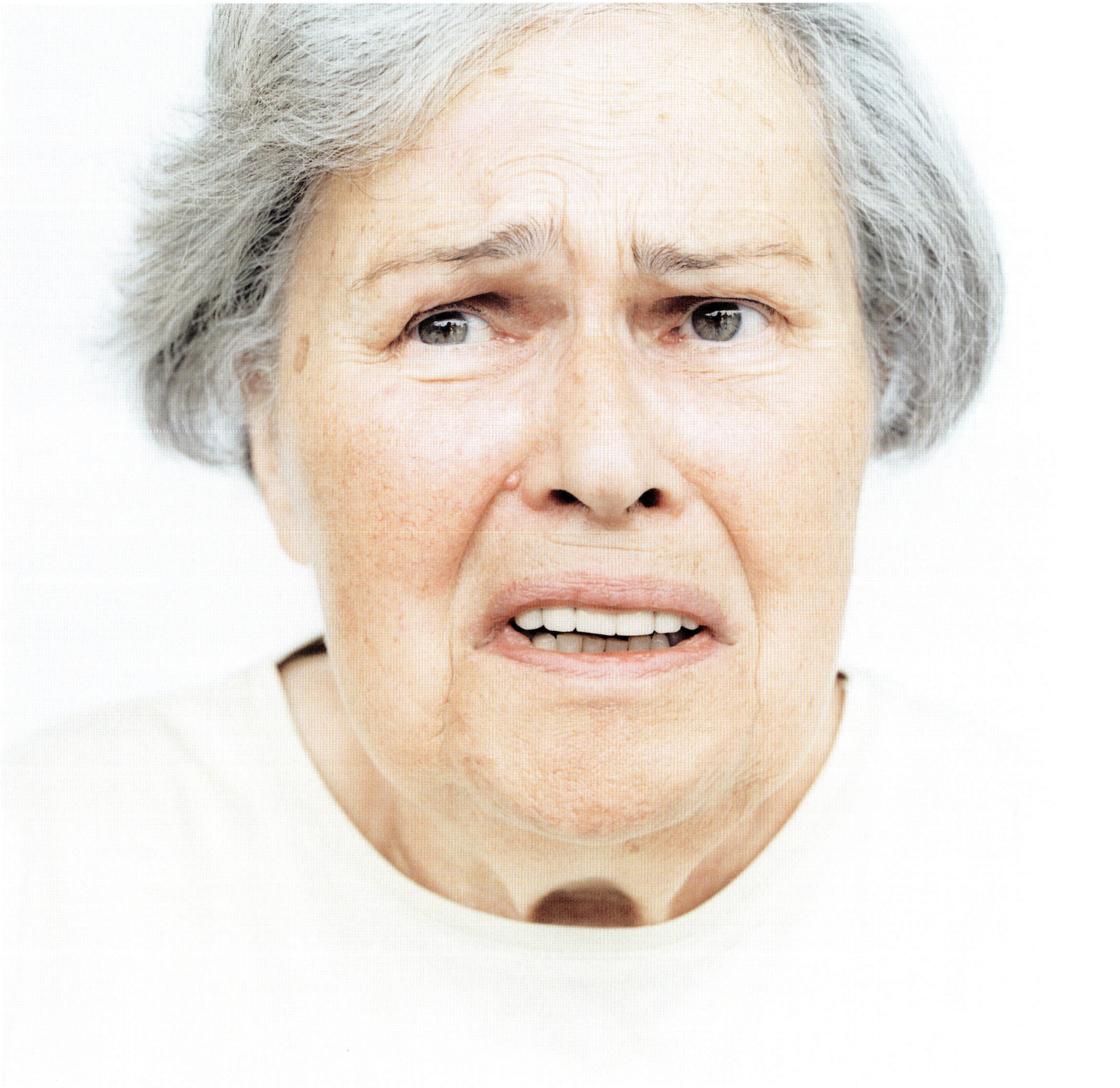

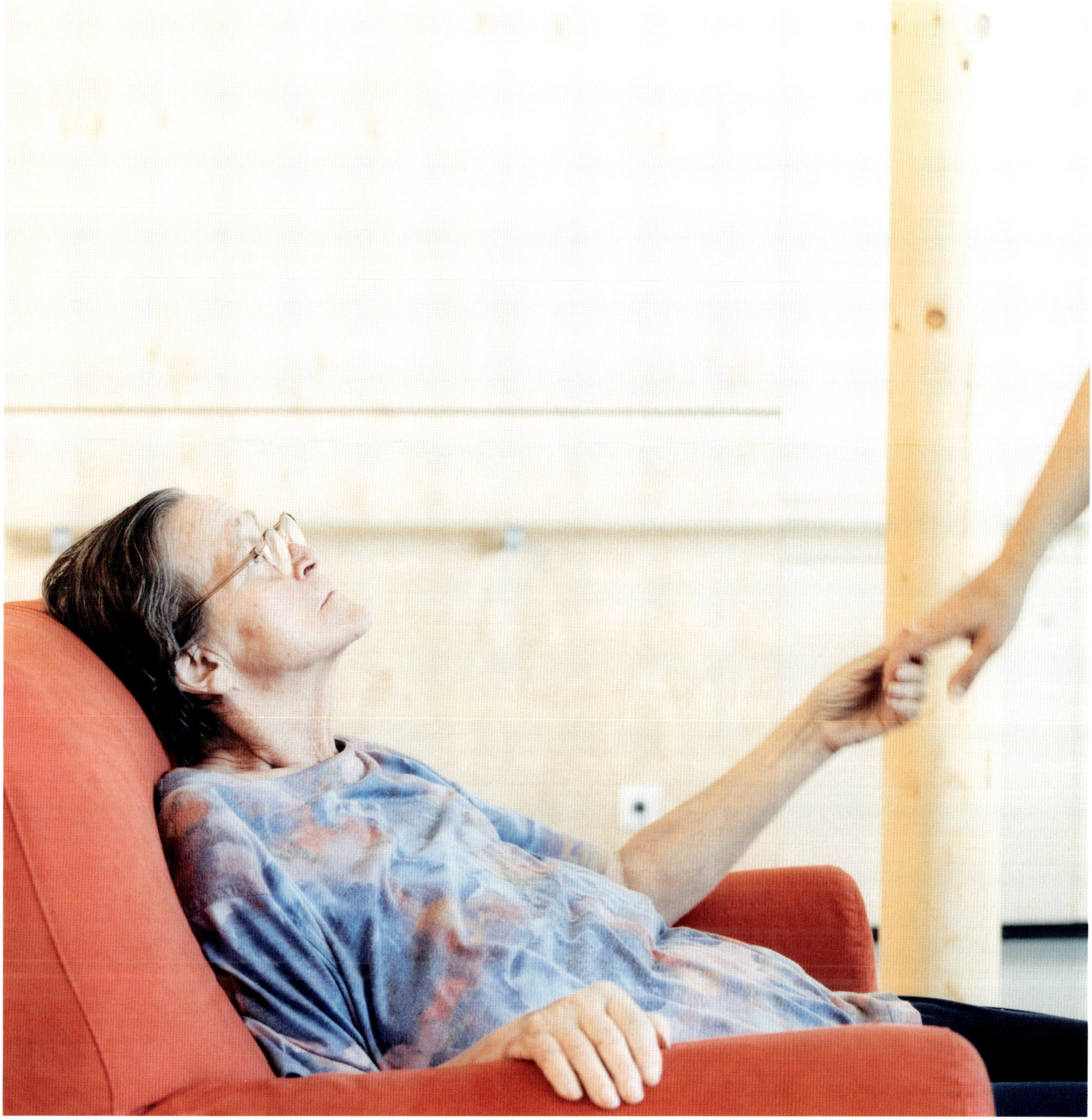

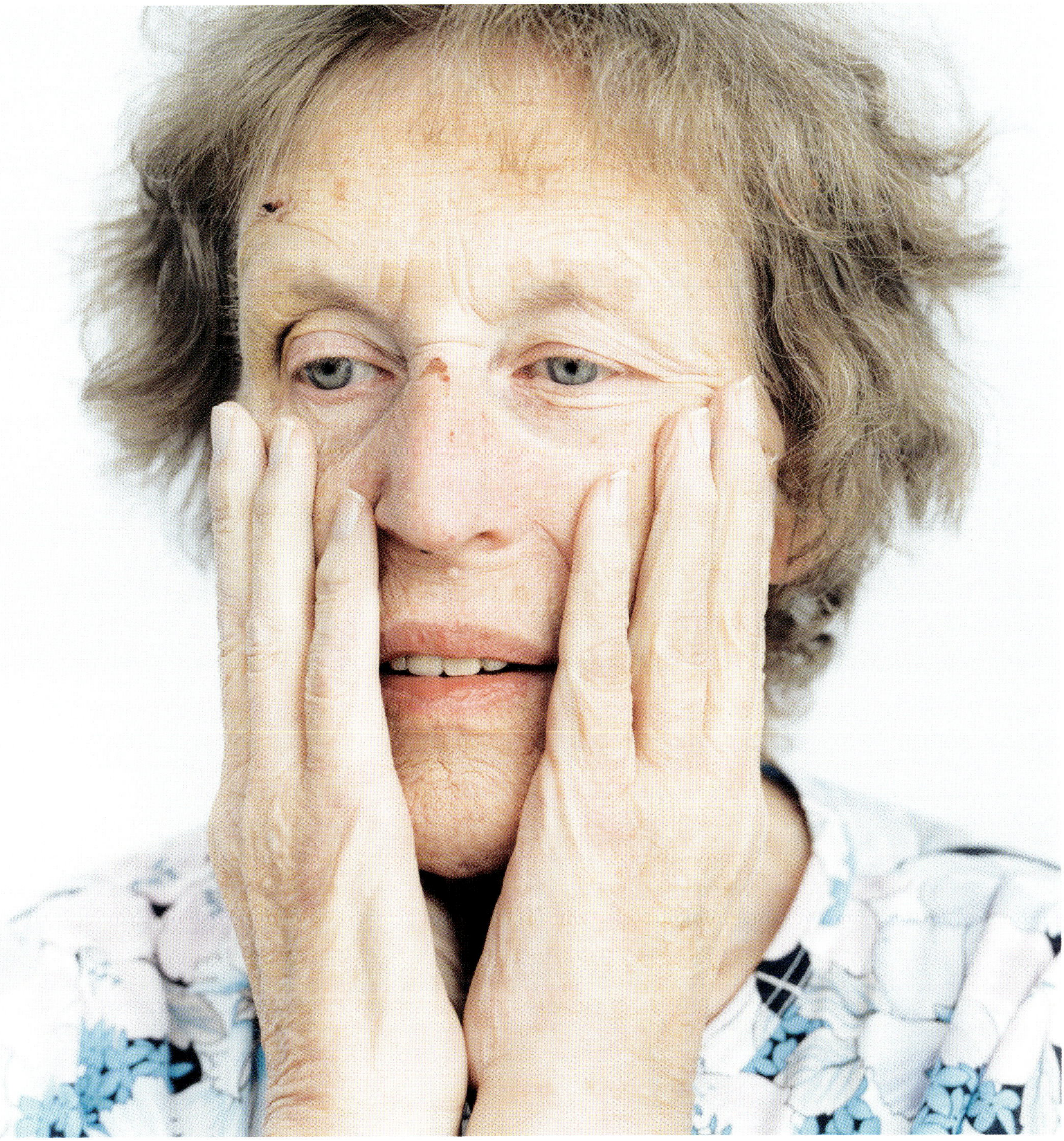

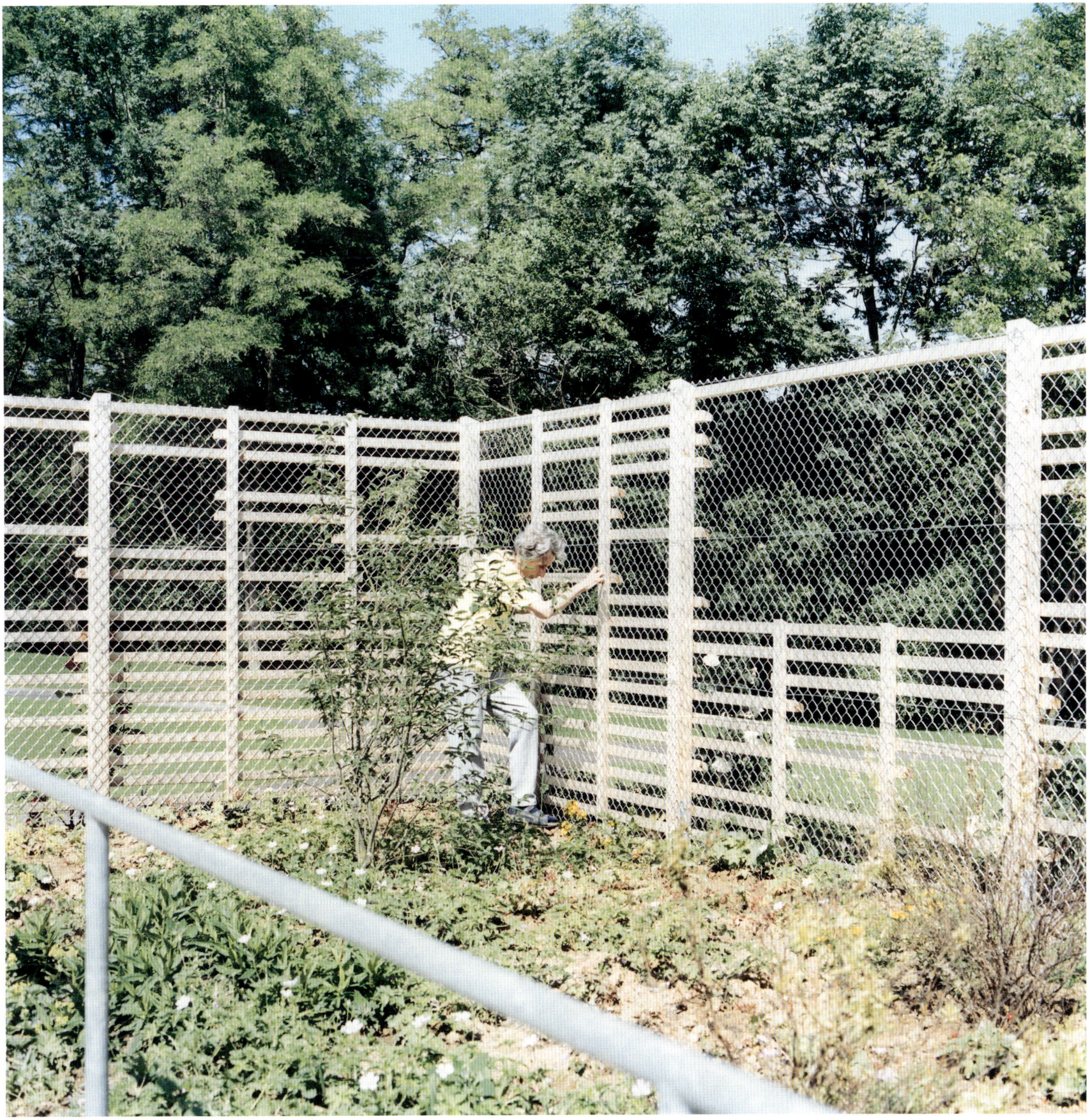

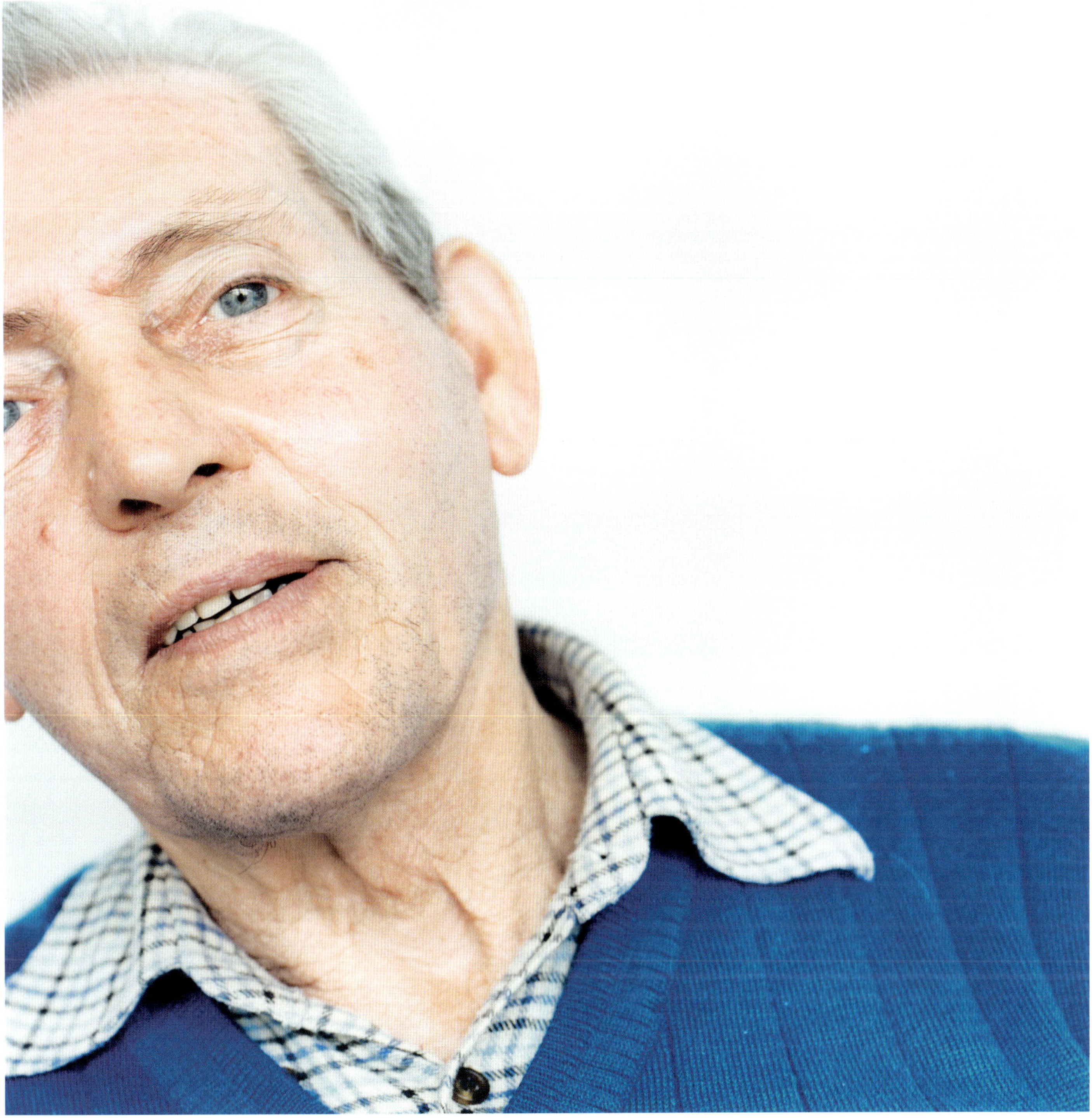

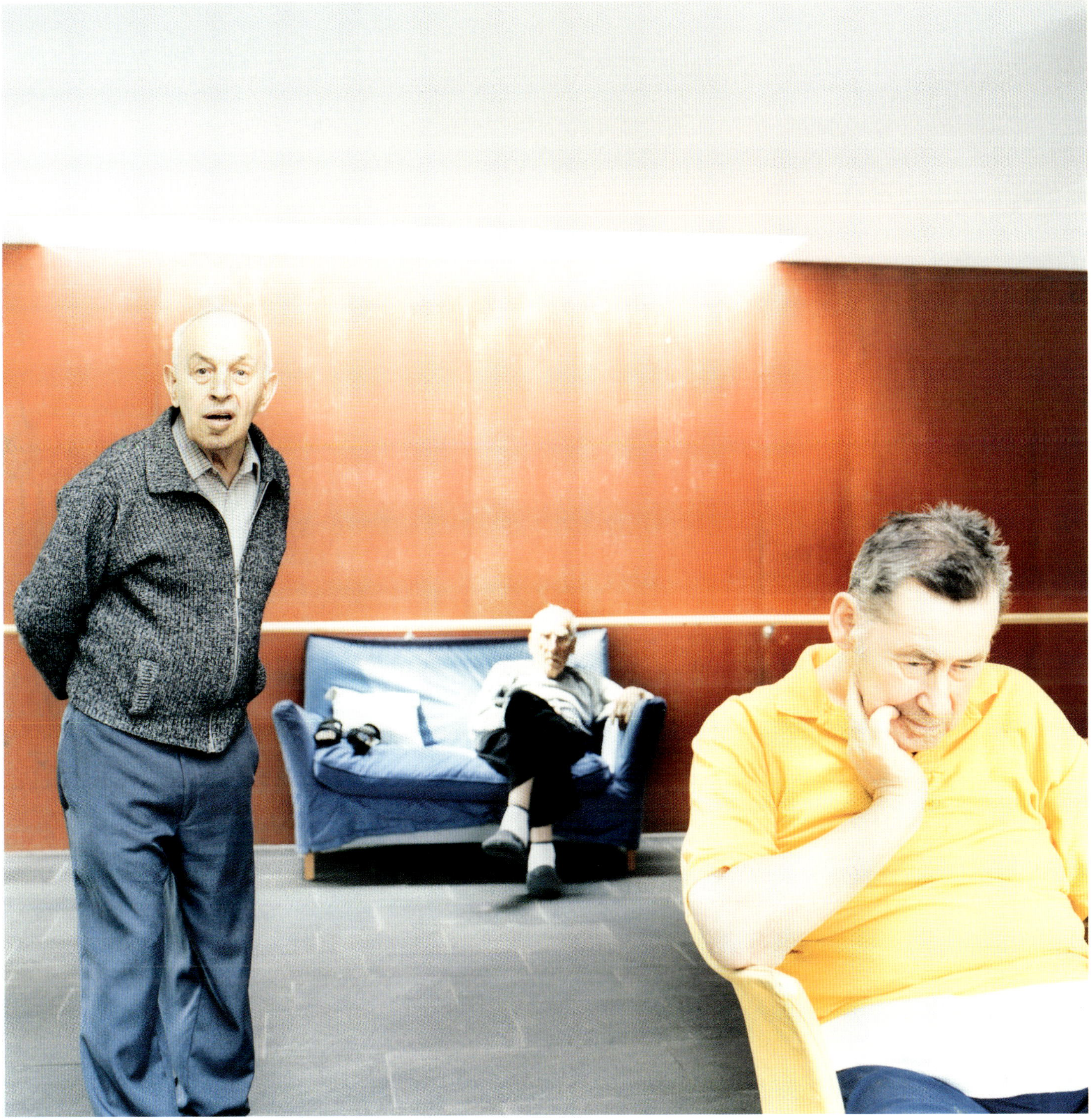

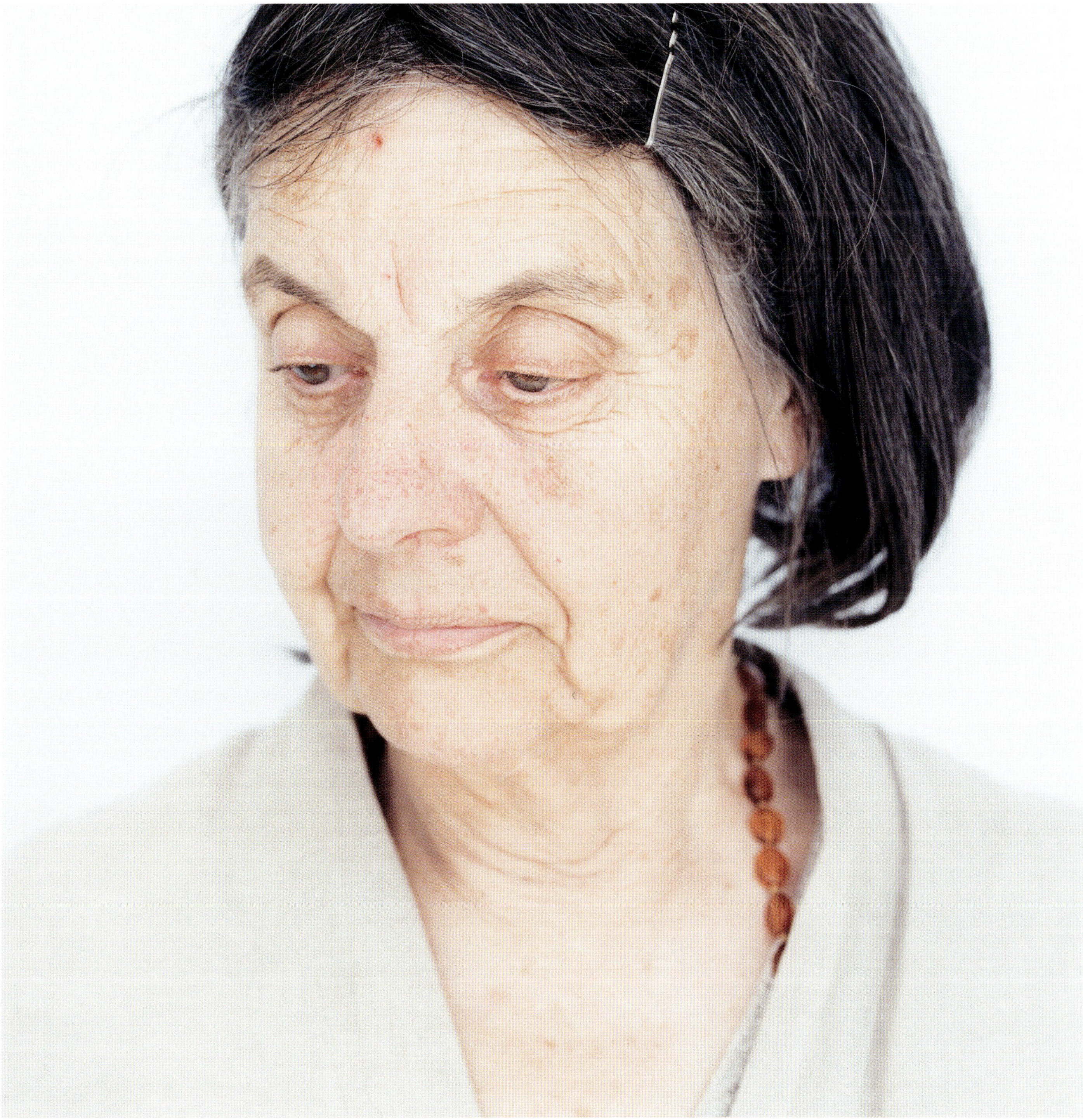

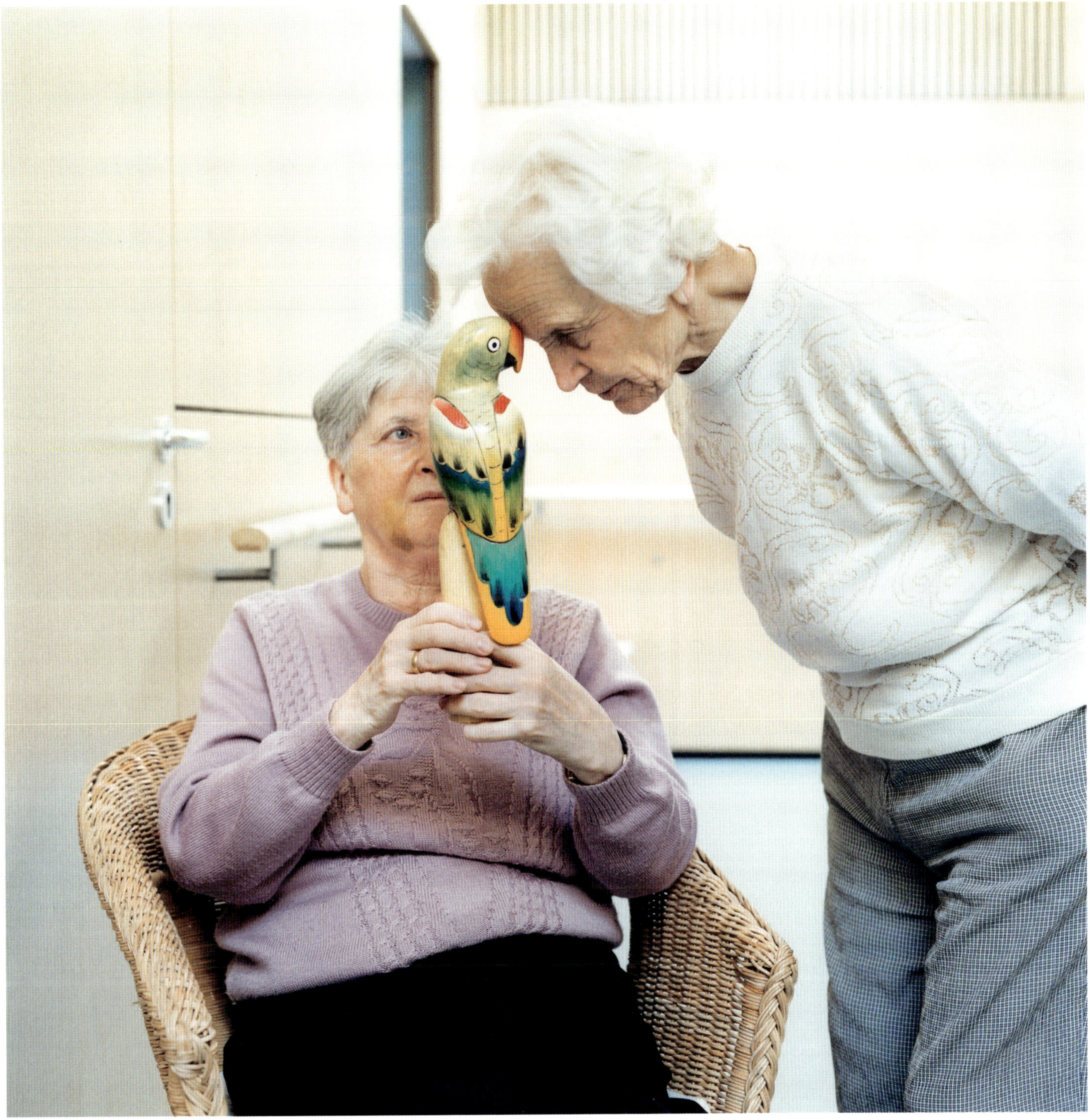

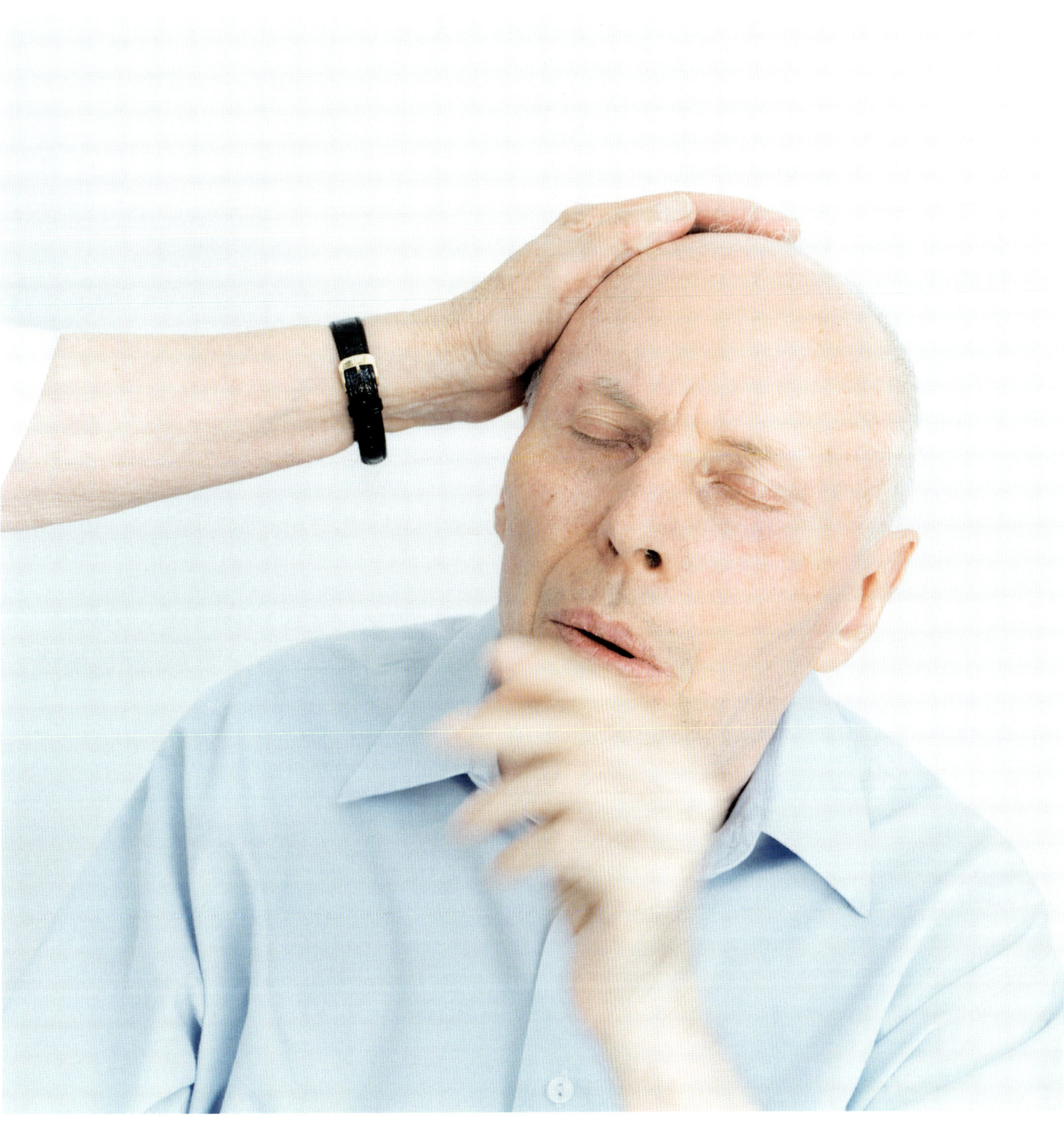

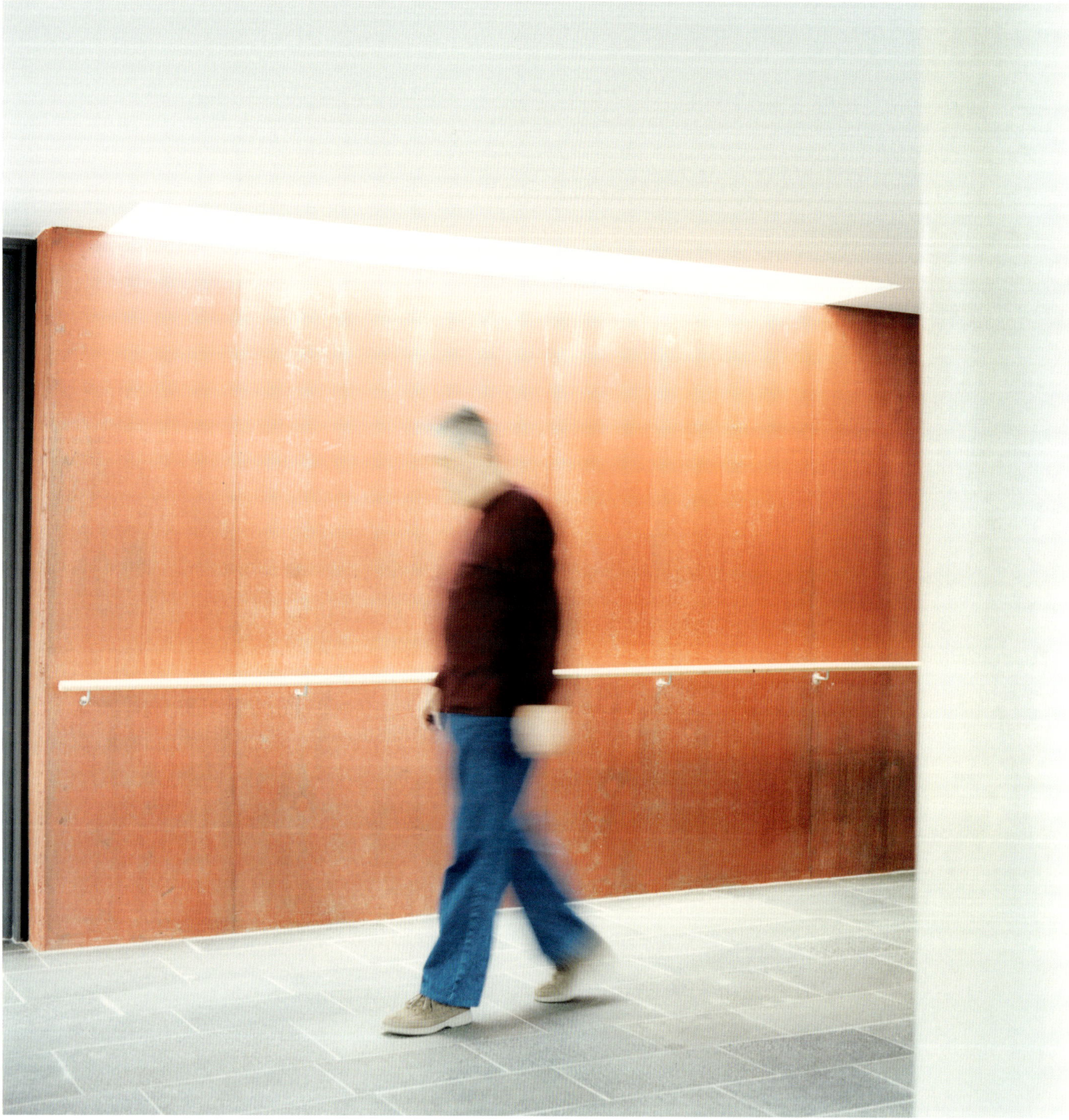

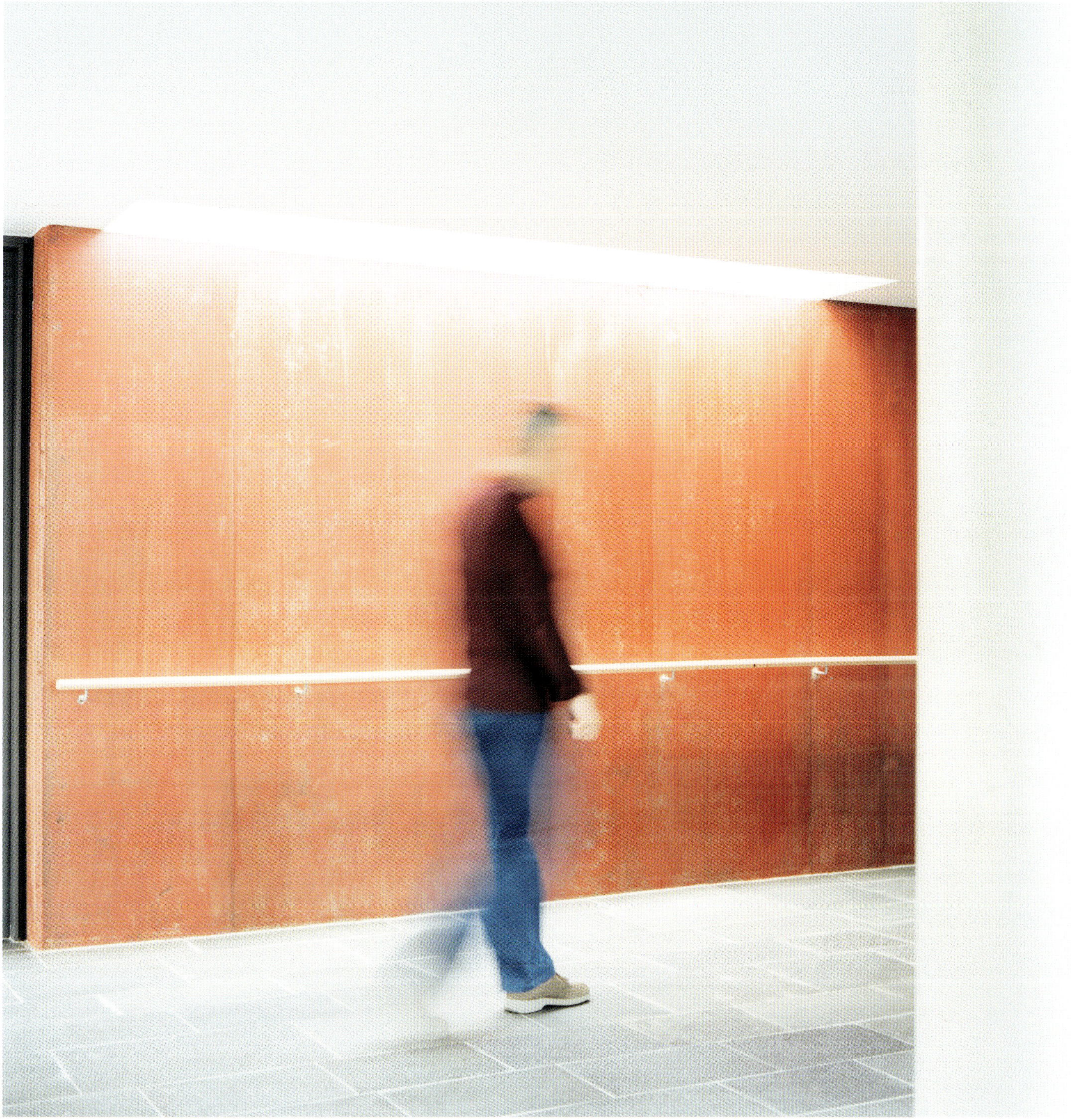

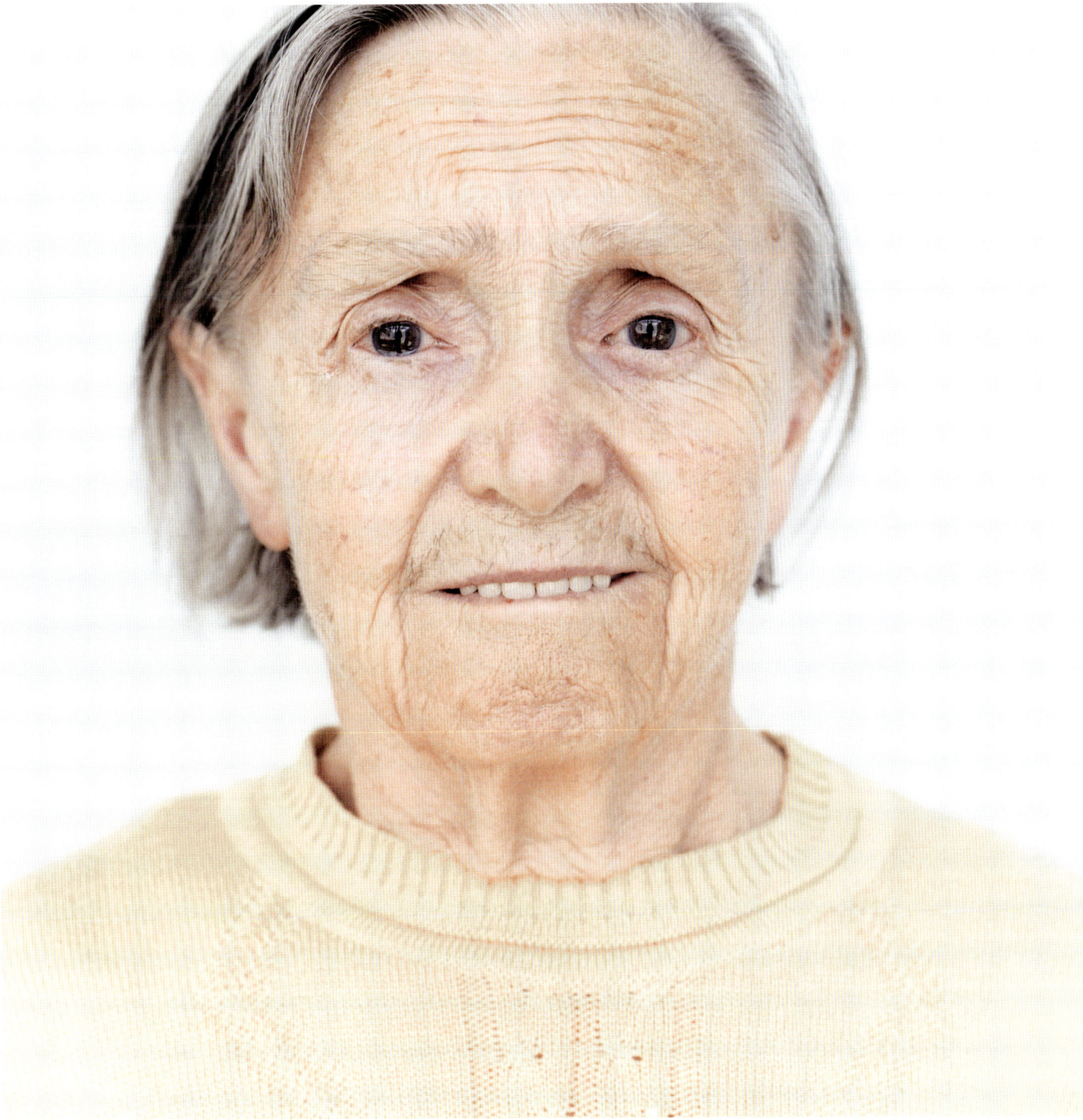

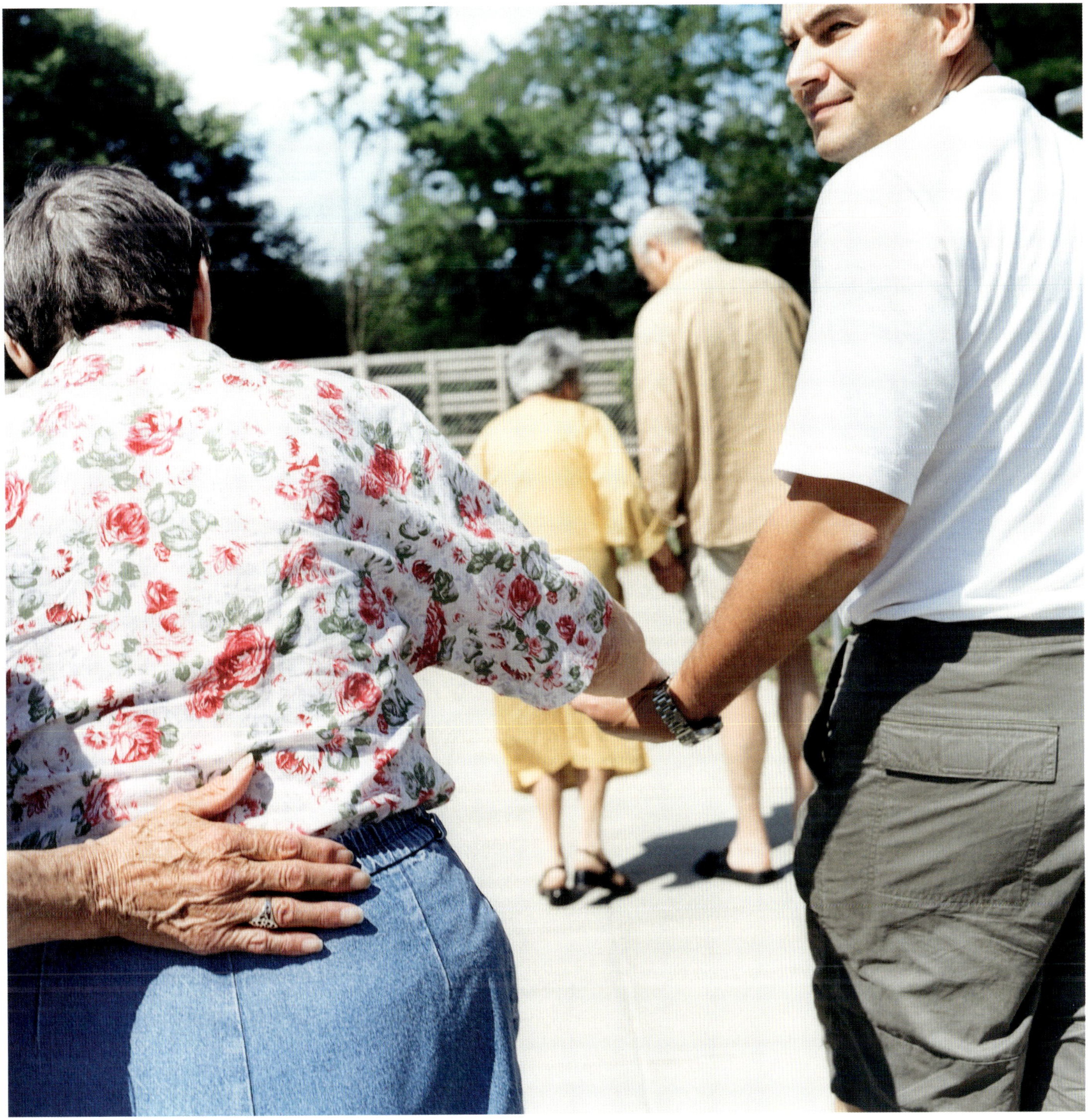

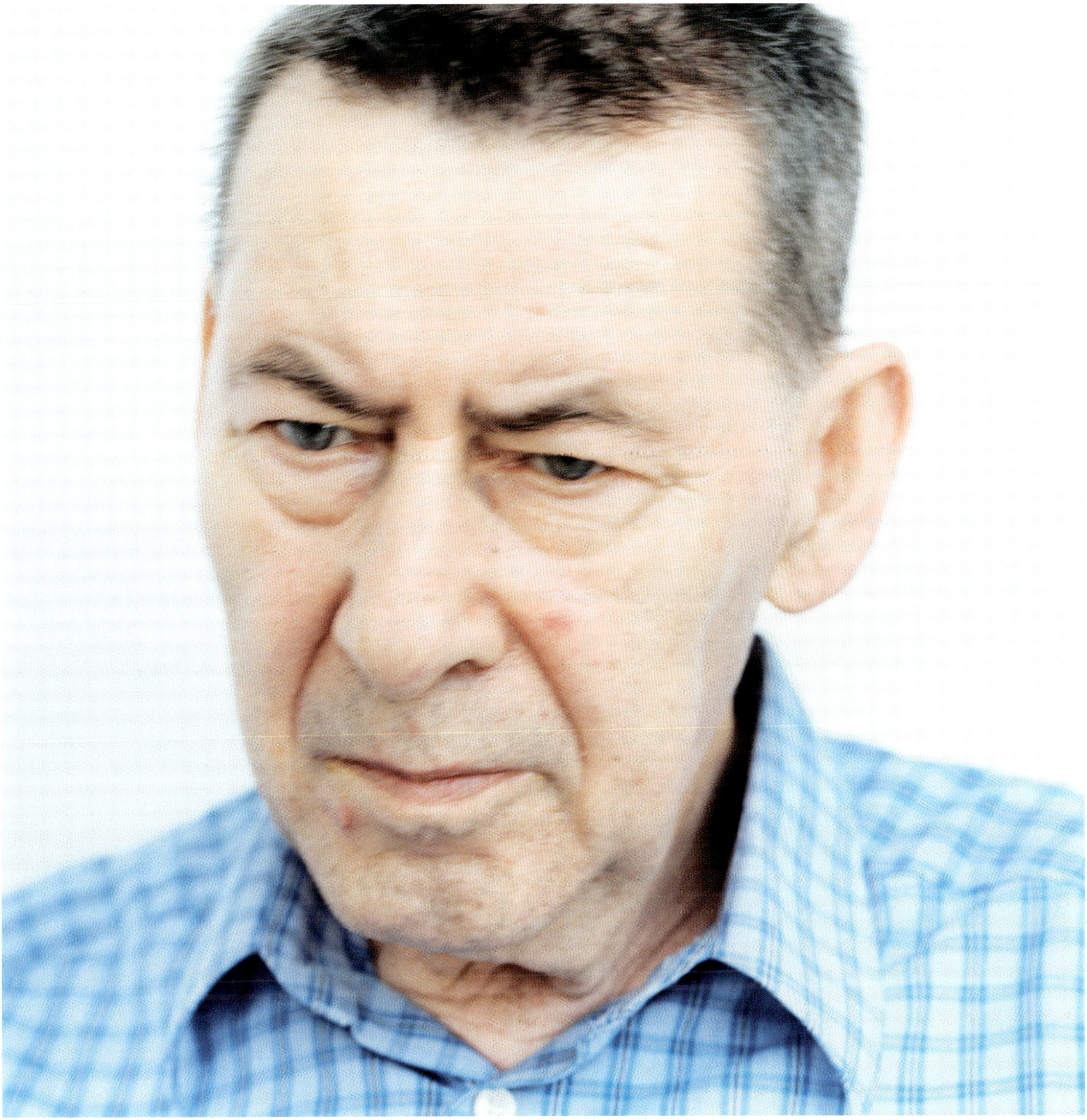

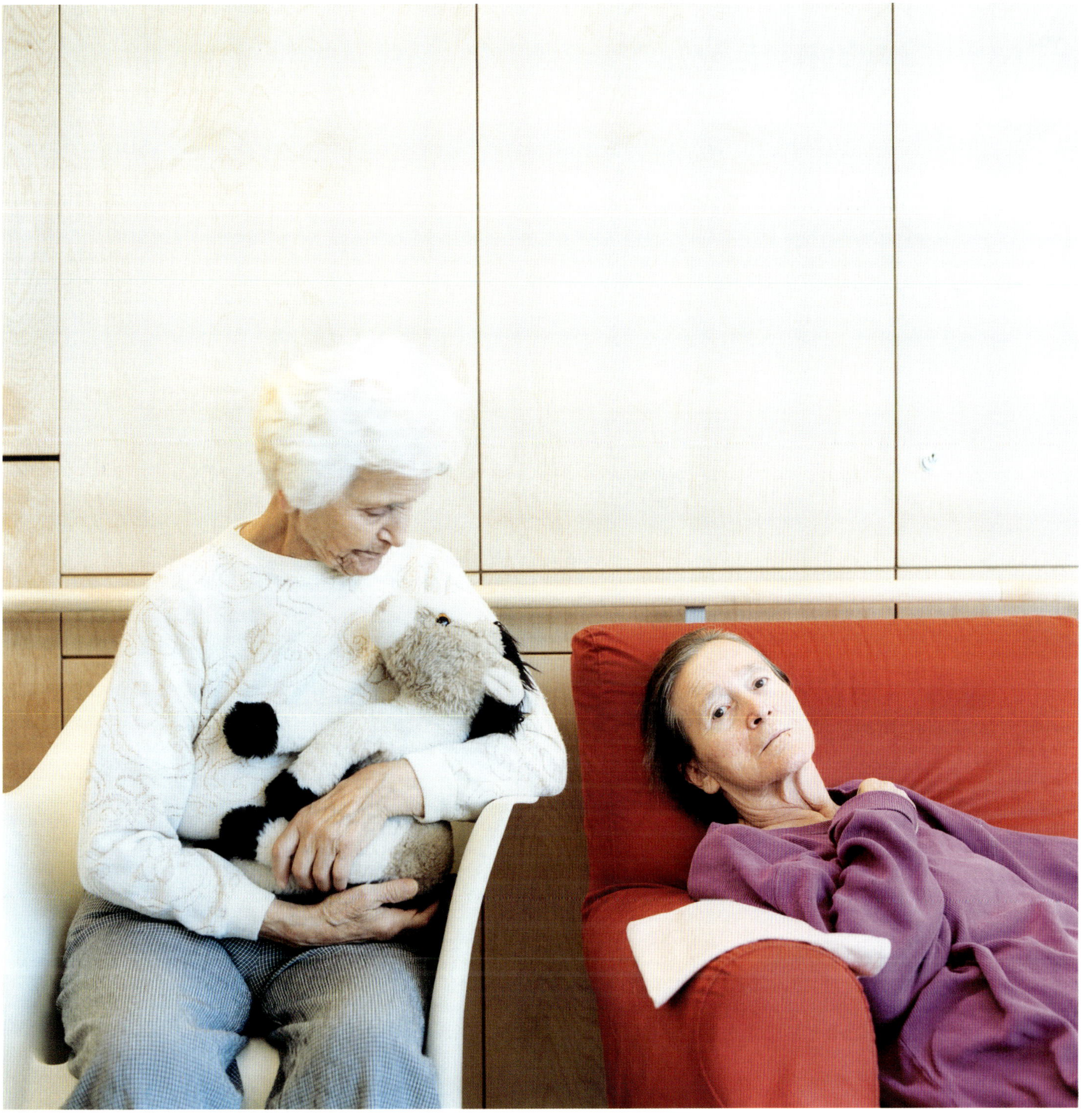

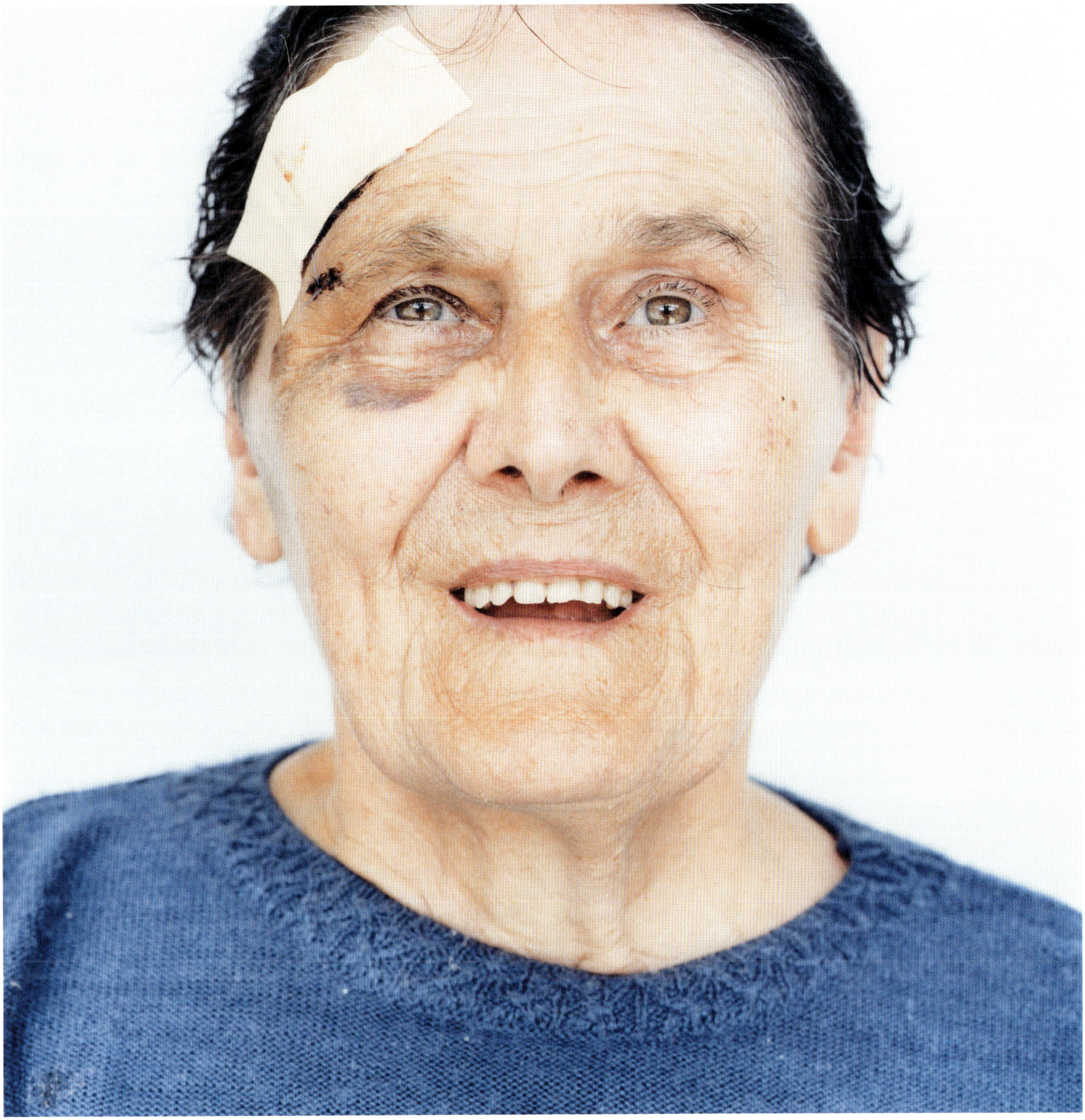

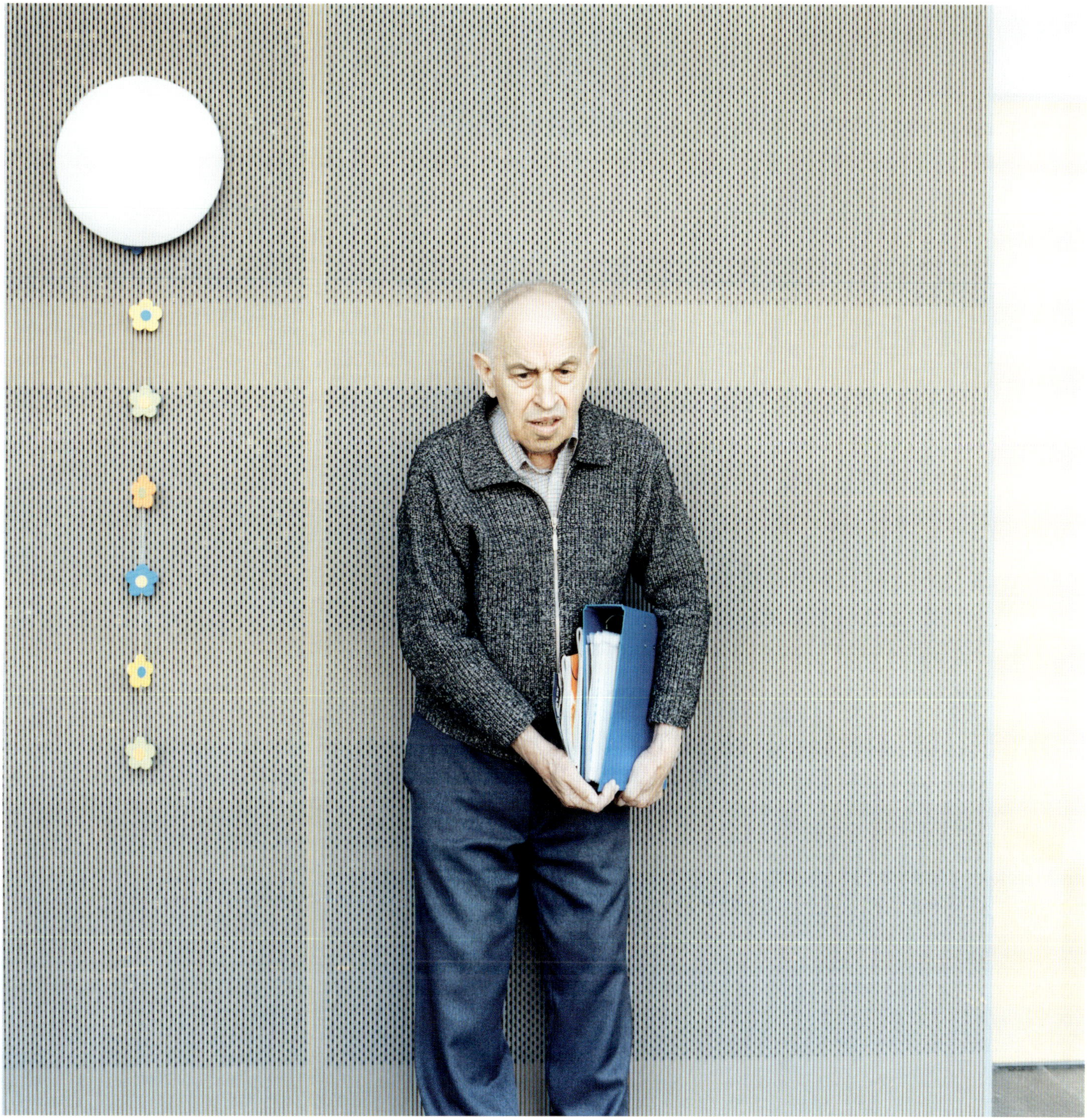

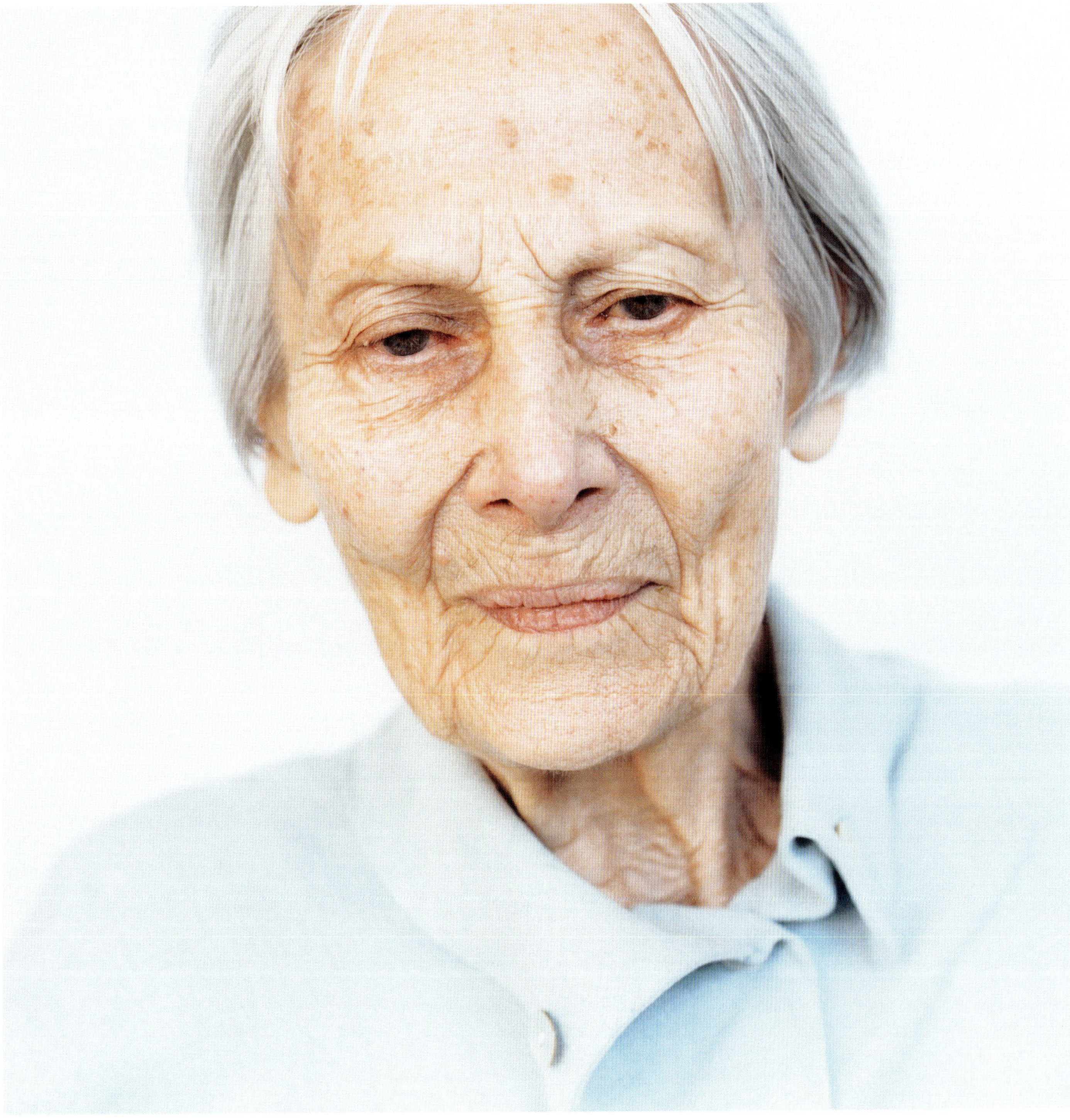

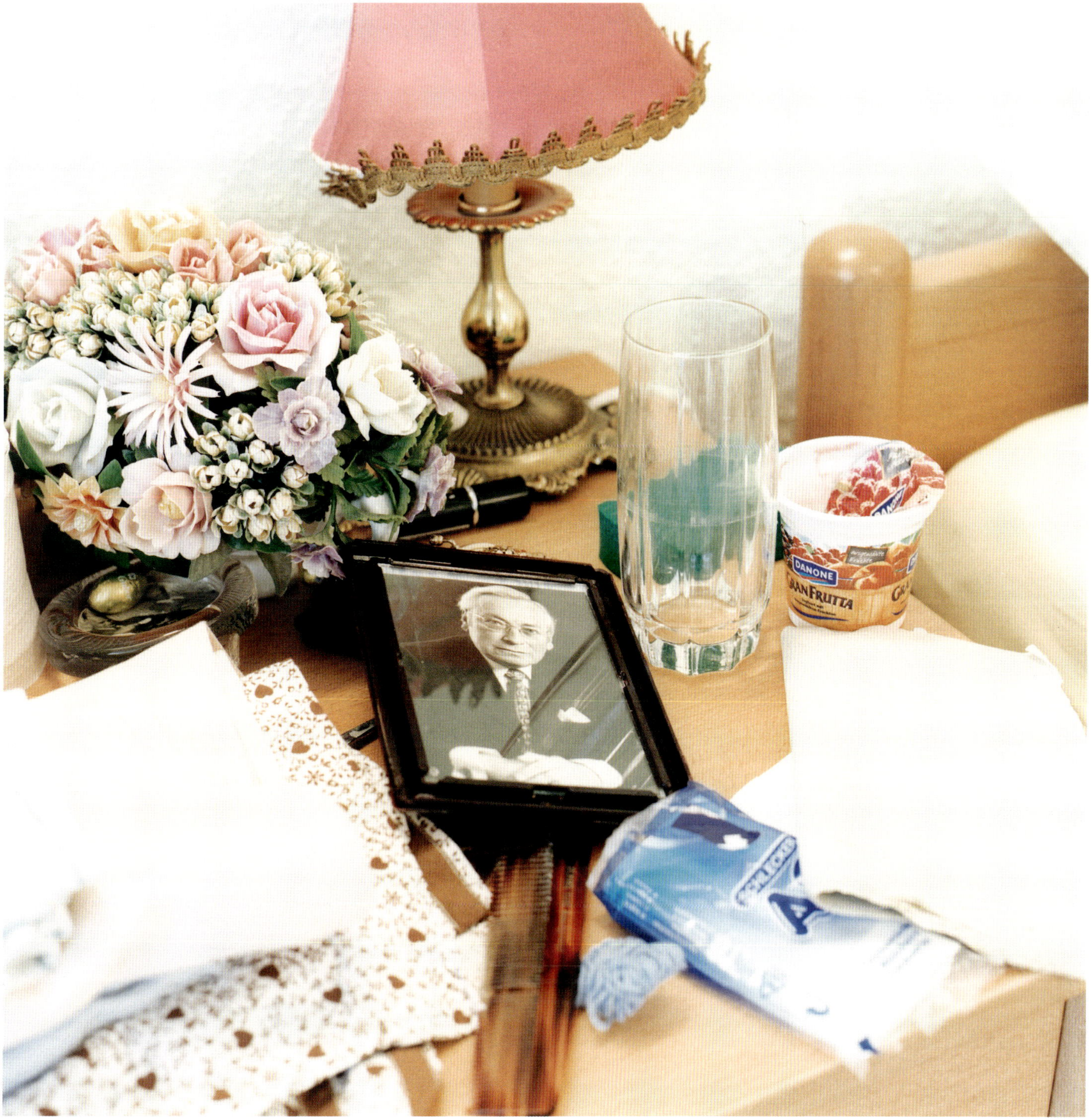
DANONE
GRAN FRUTTA

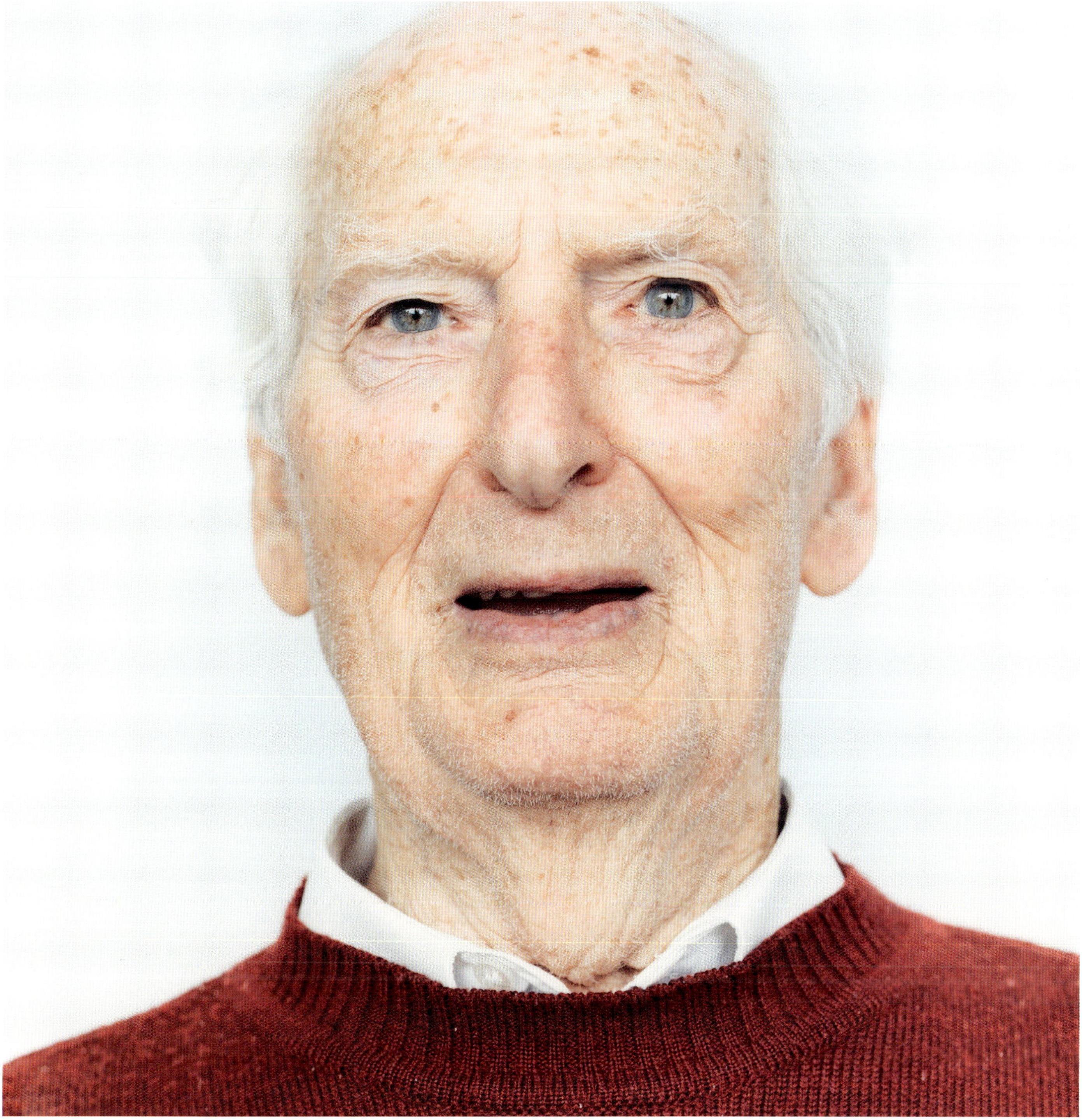

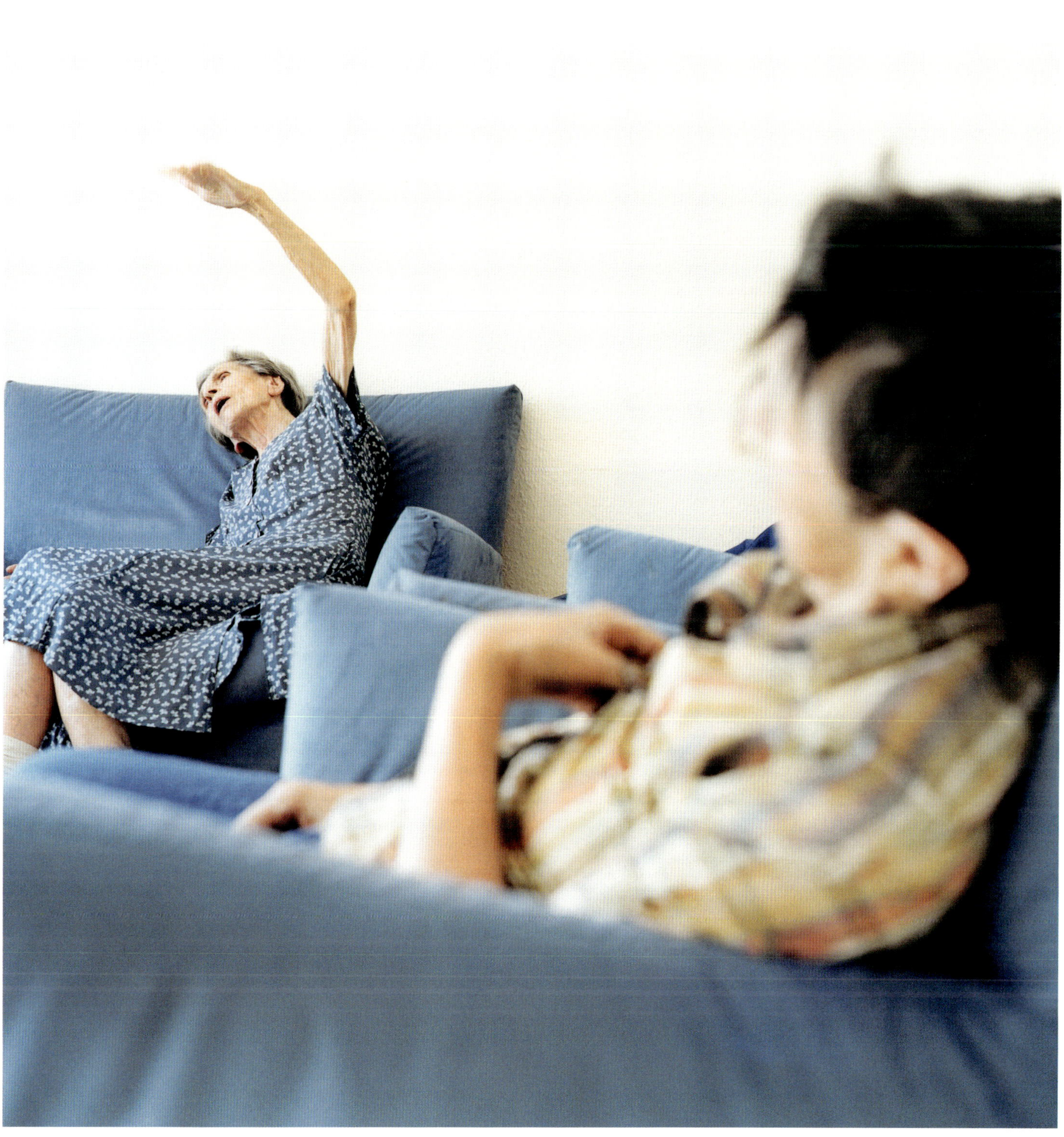

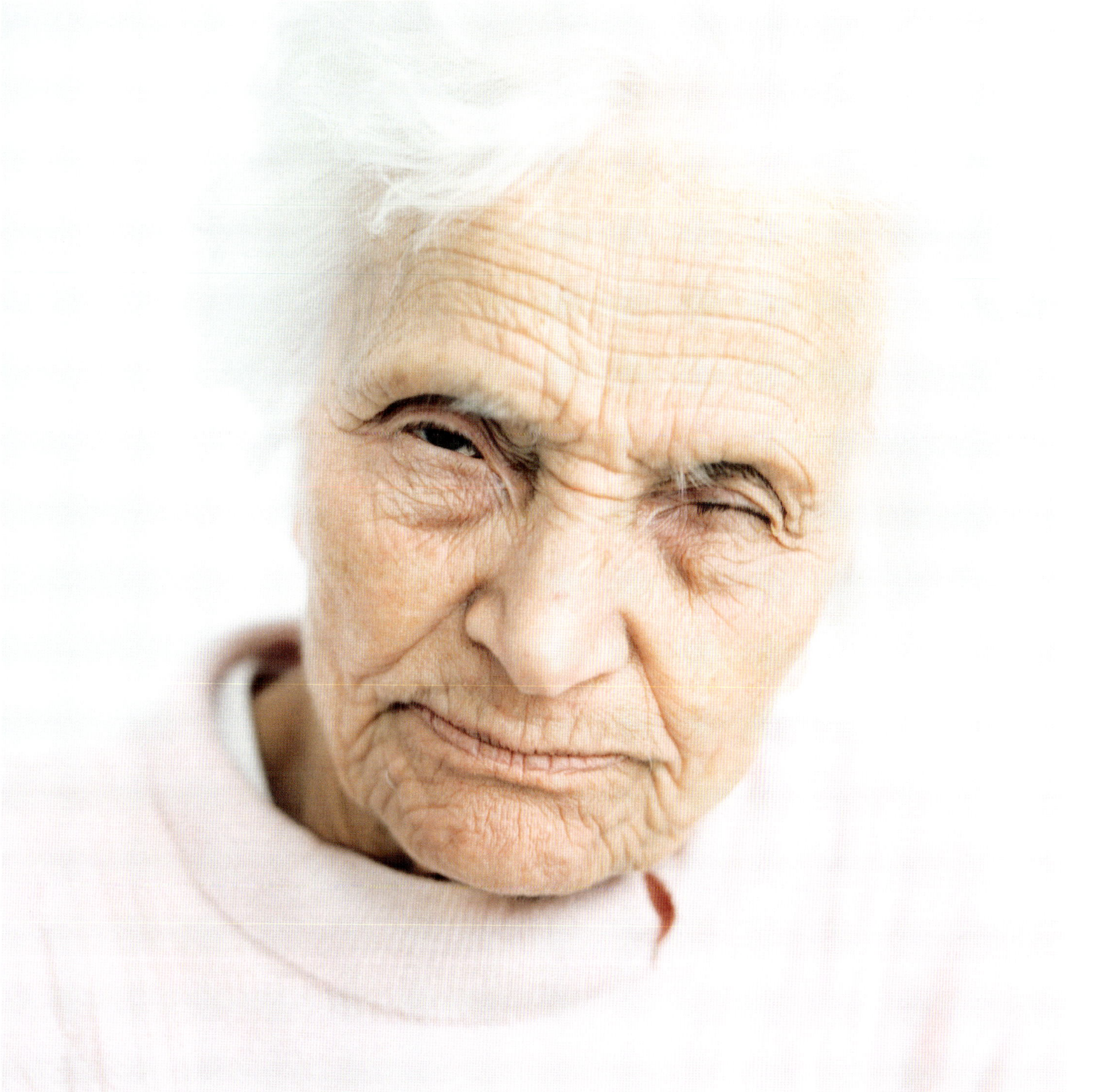

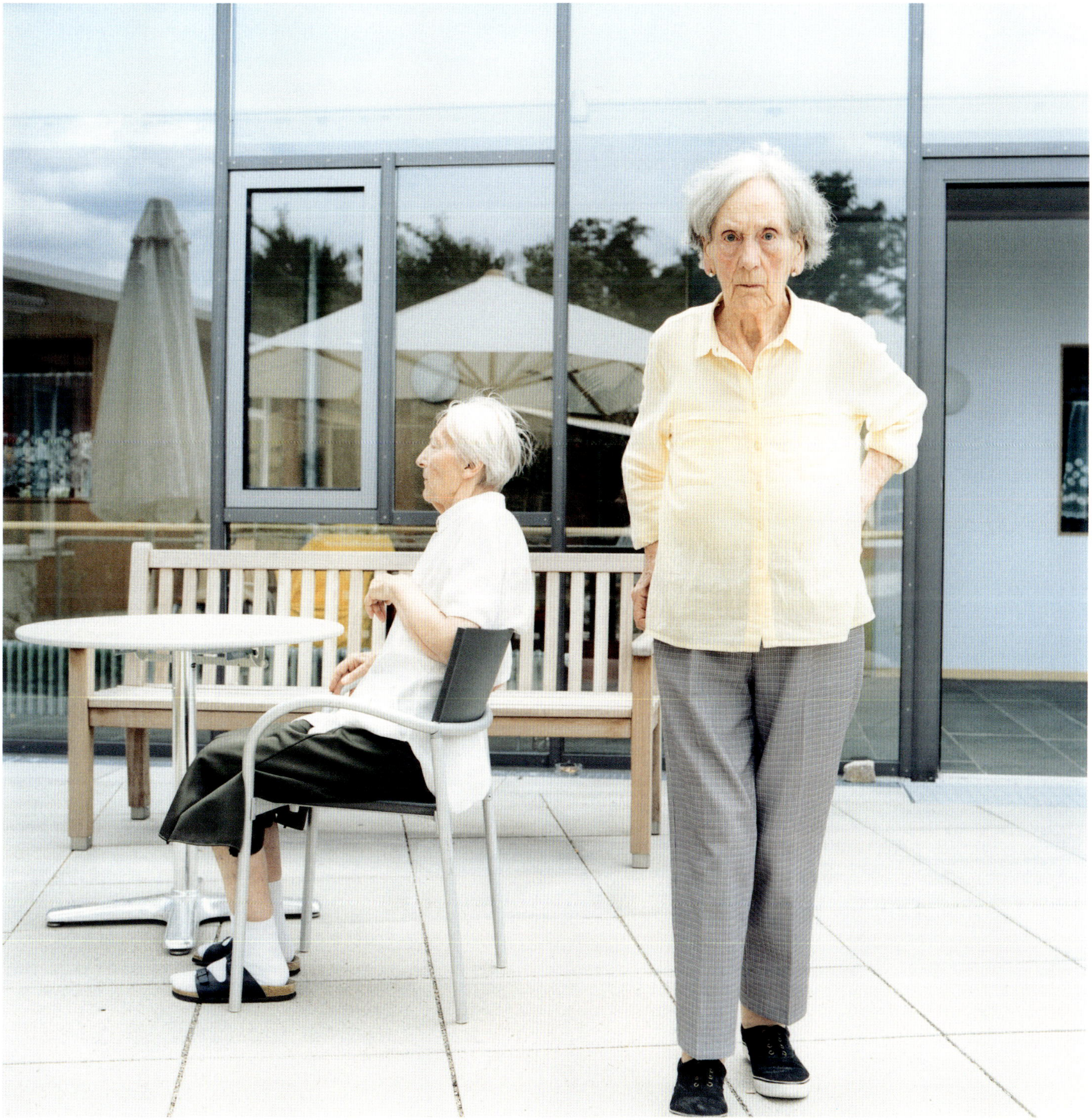

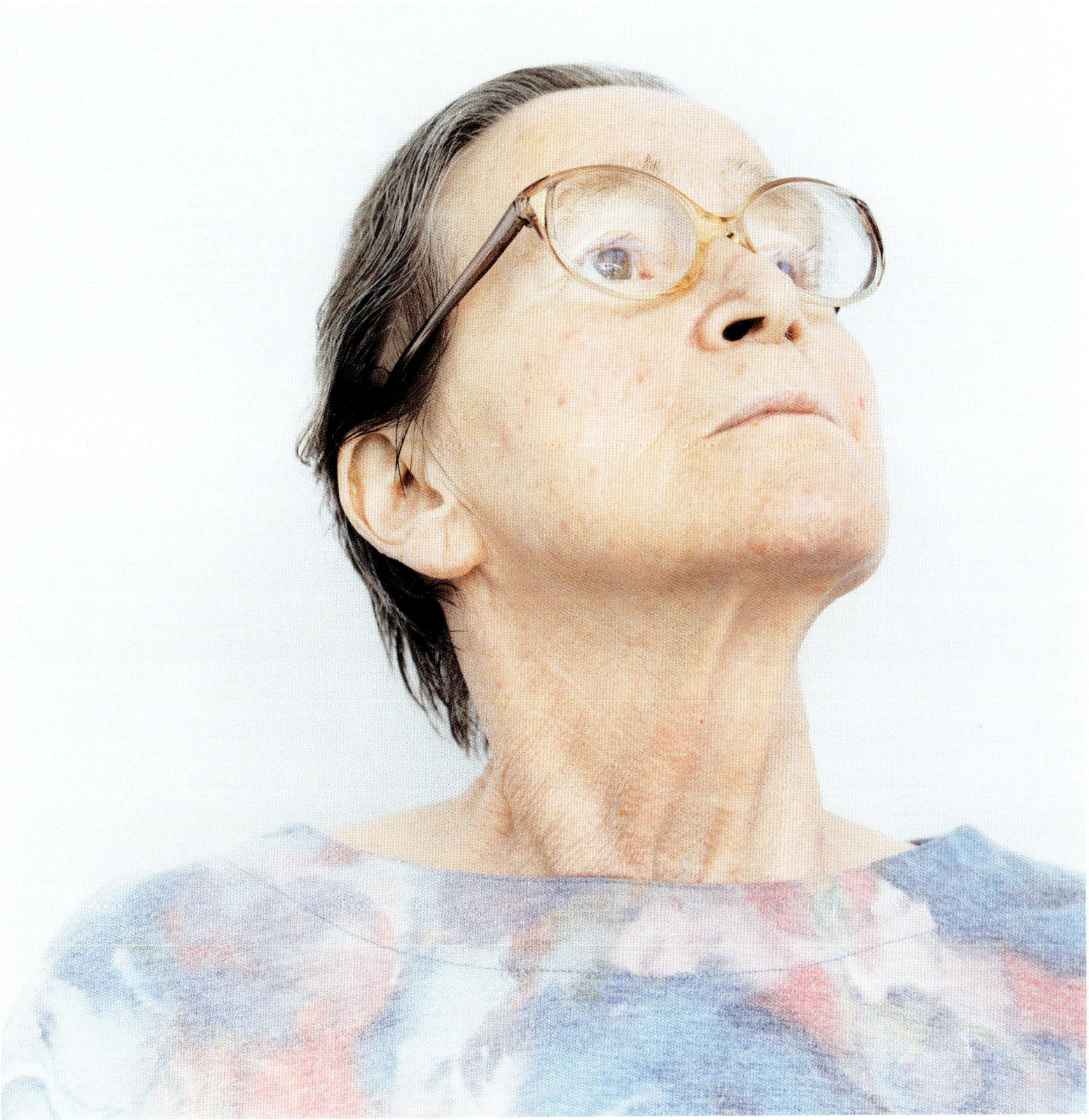

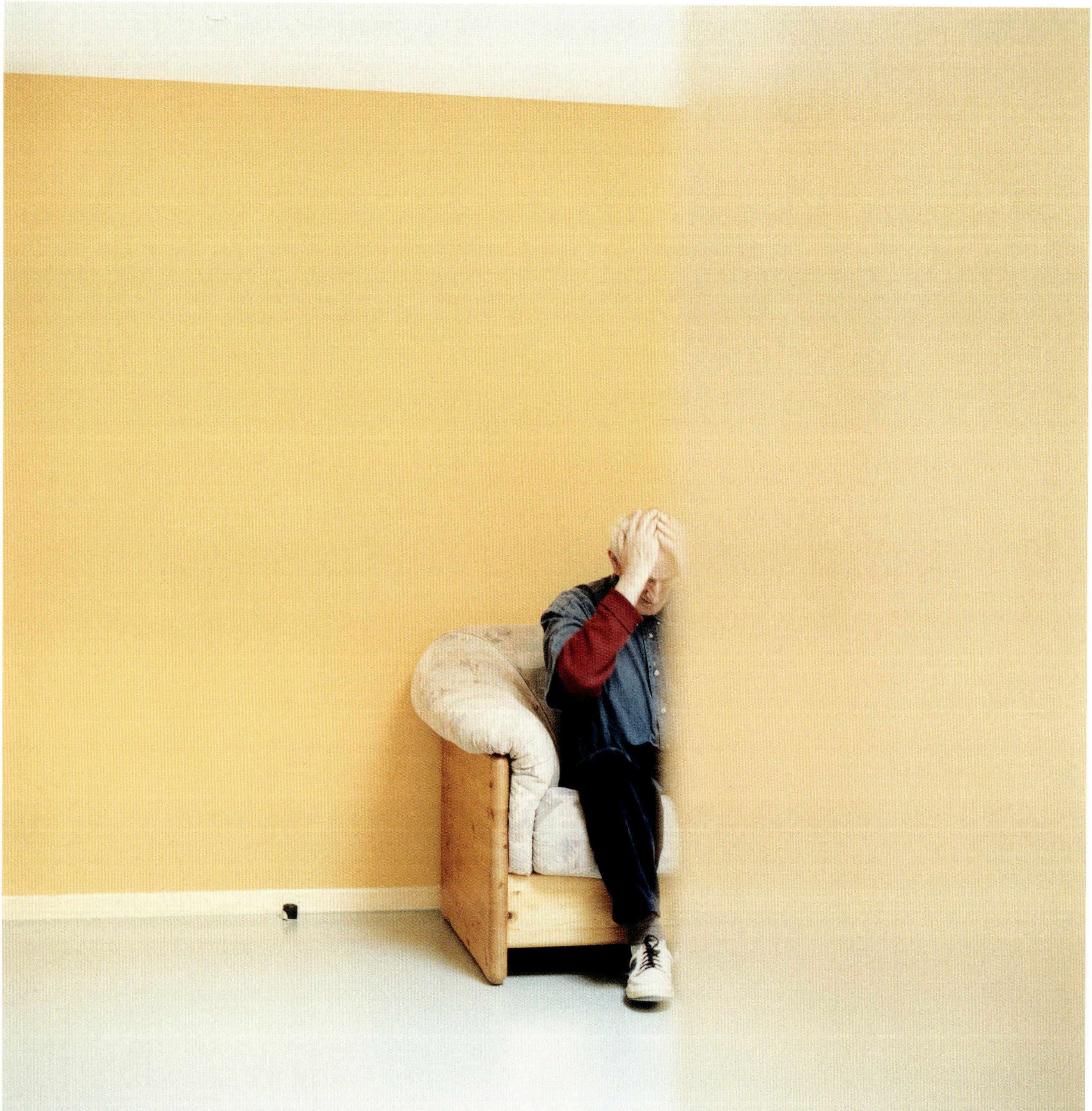

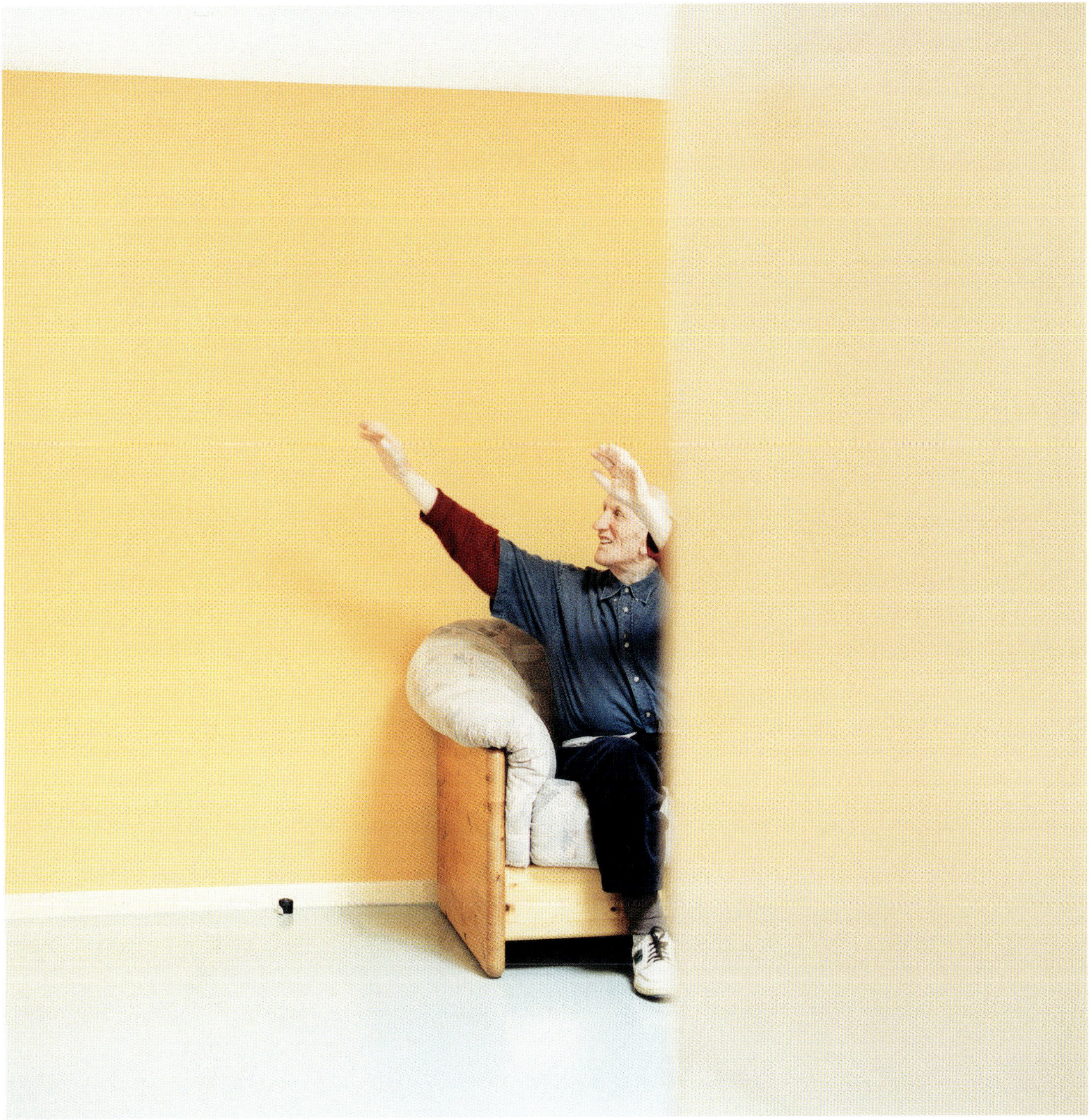

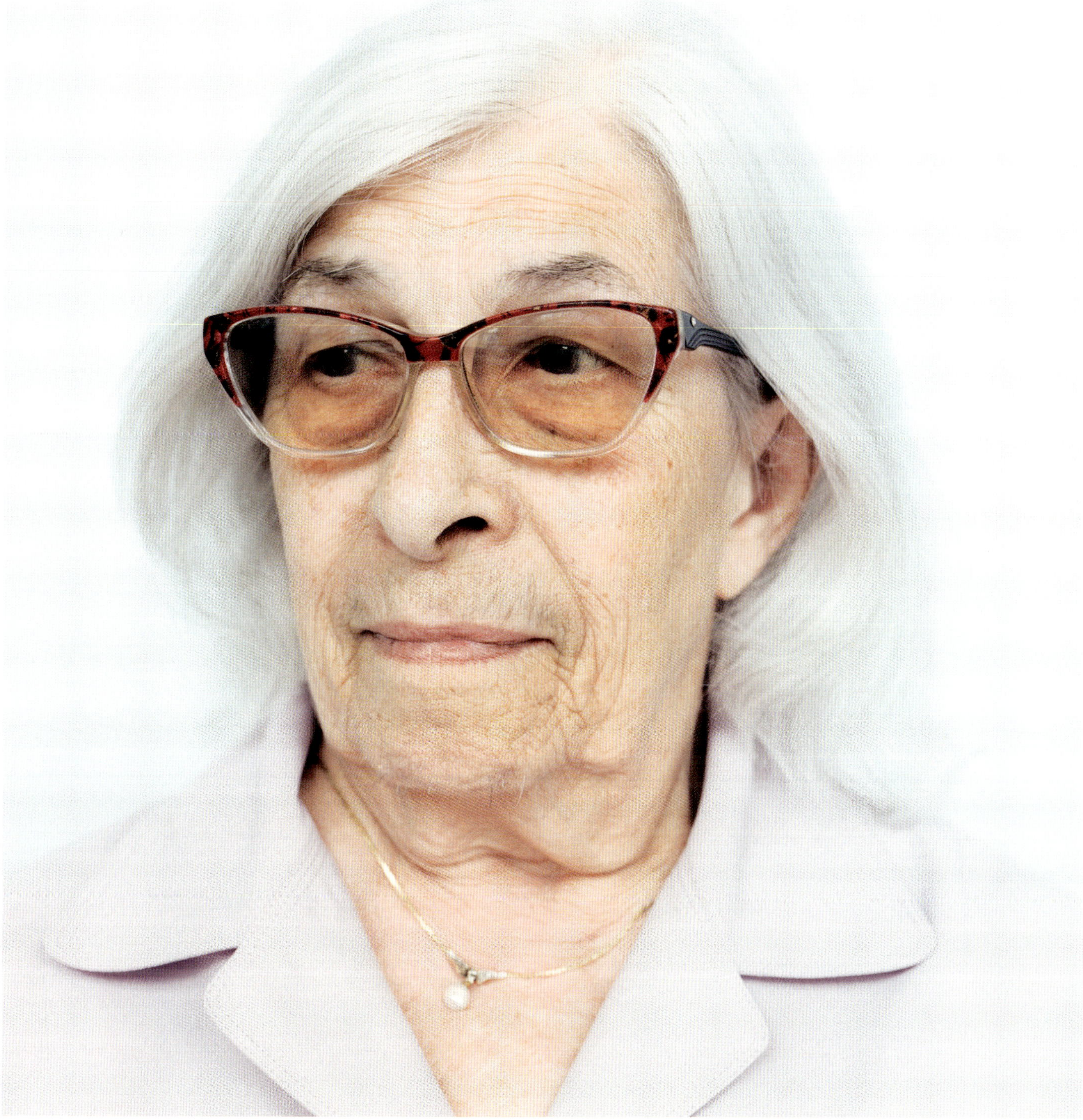

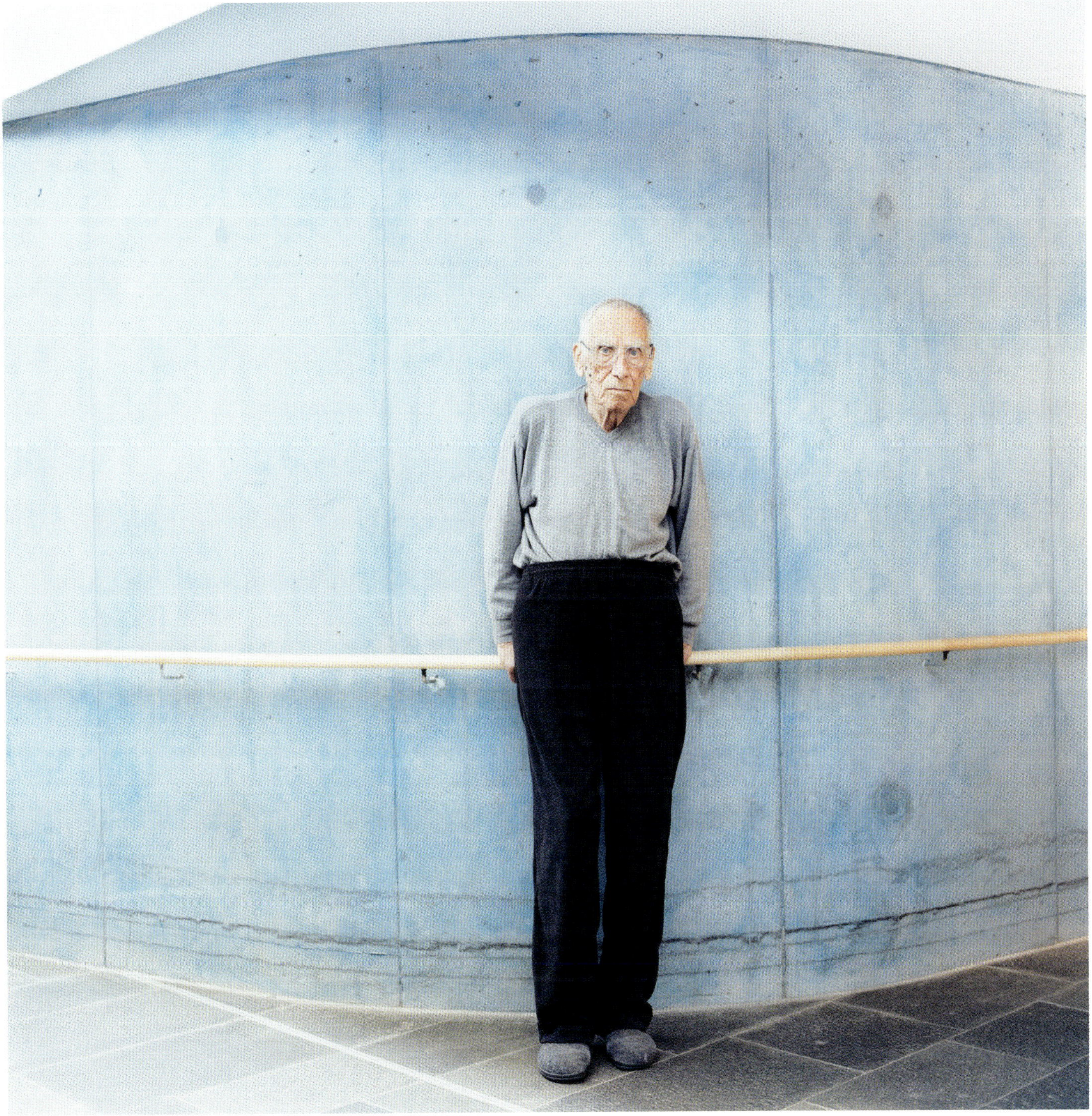

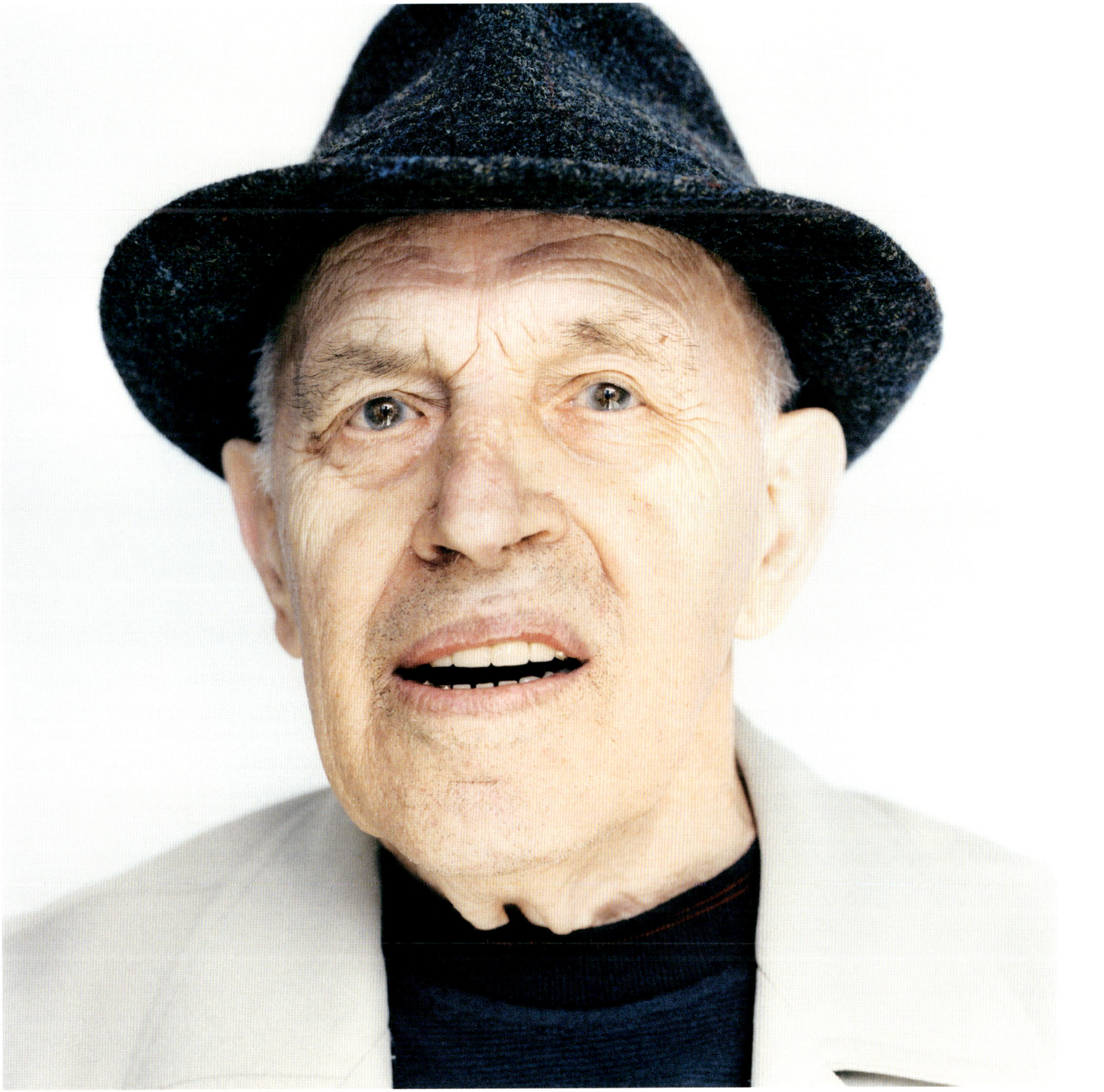

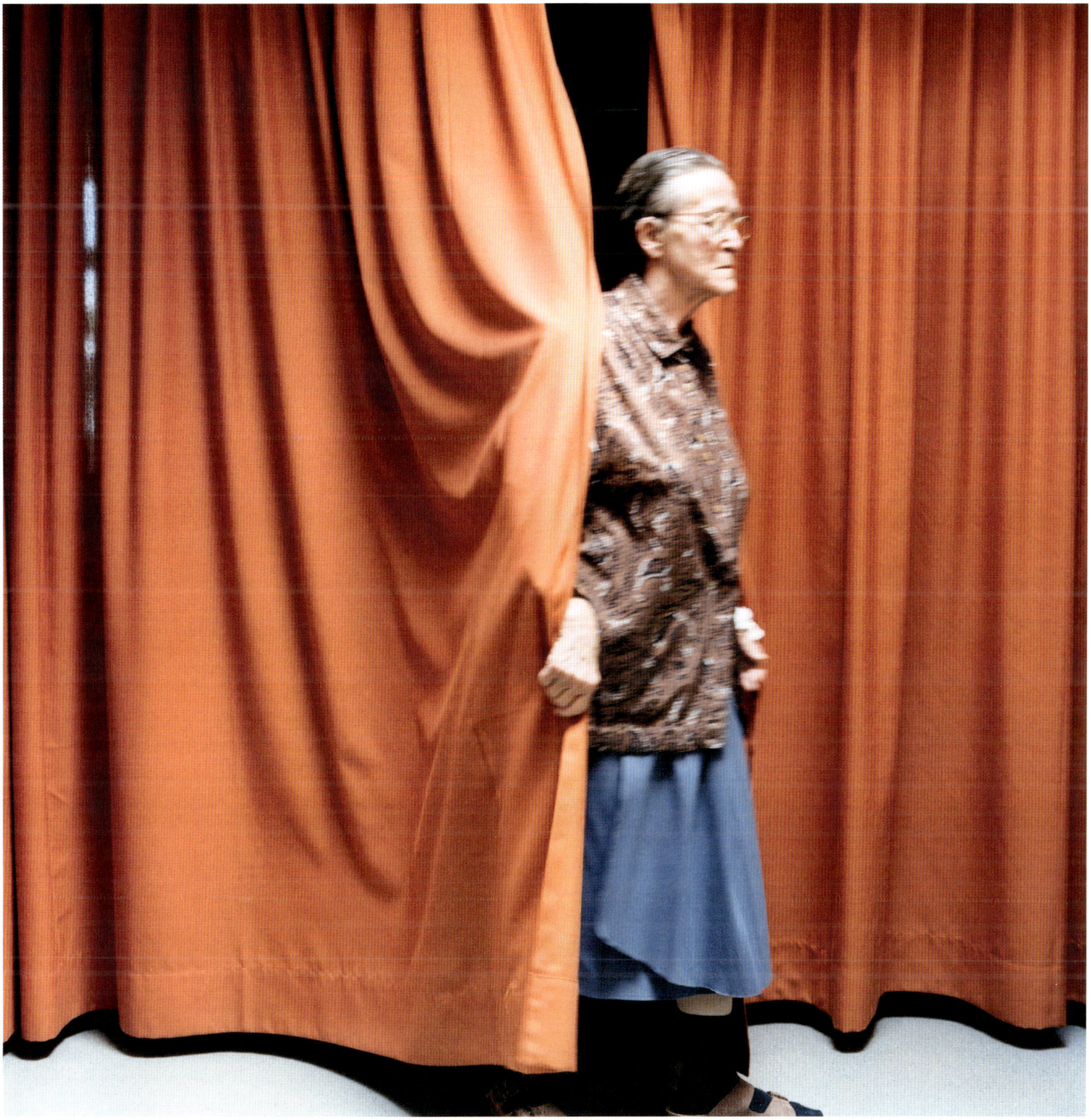

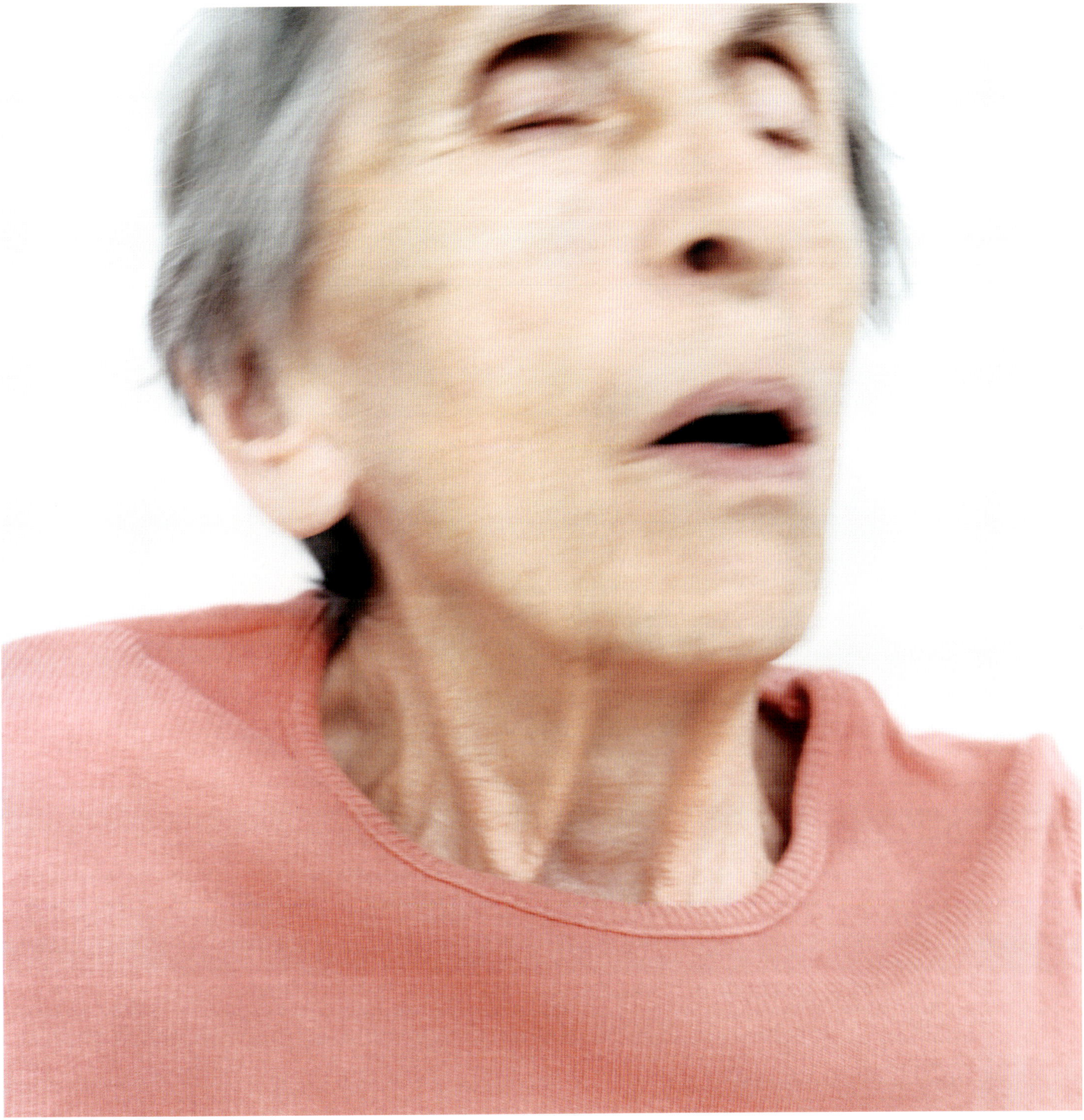

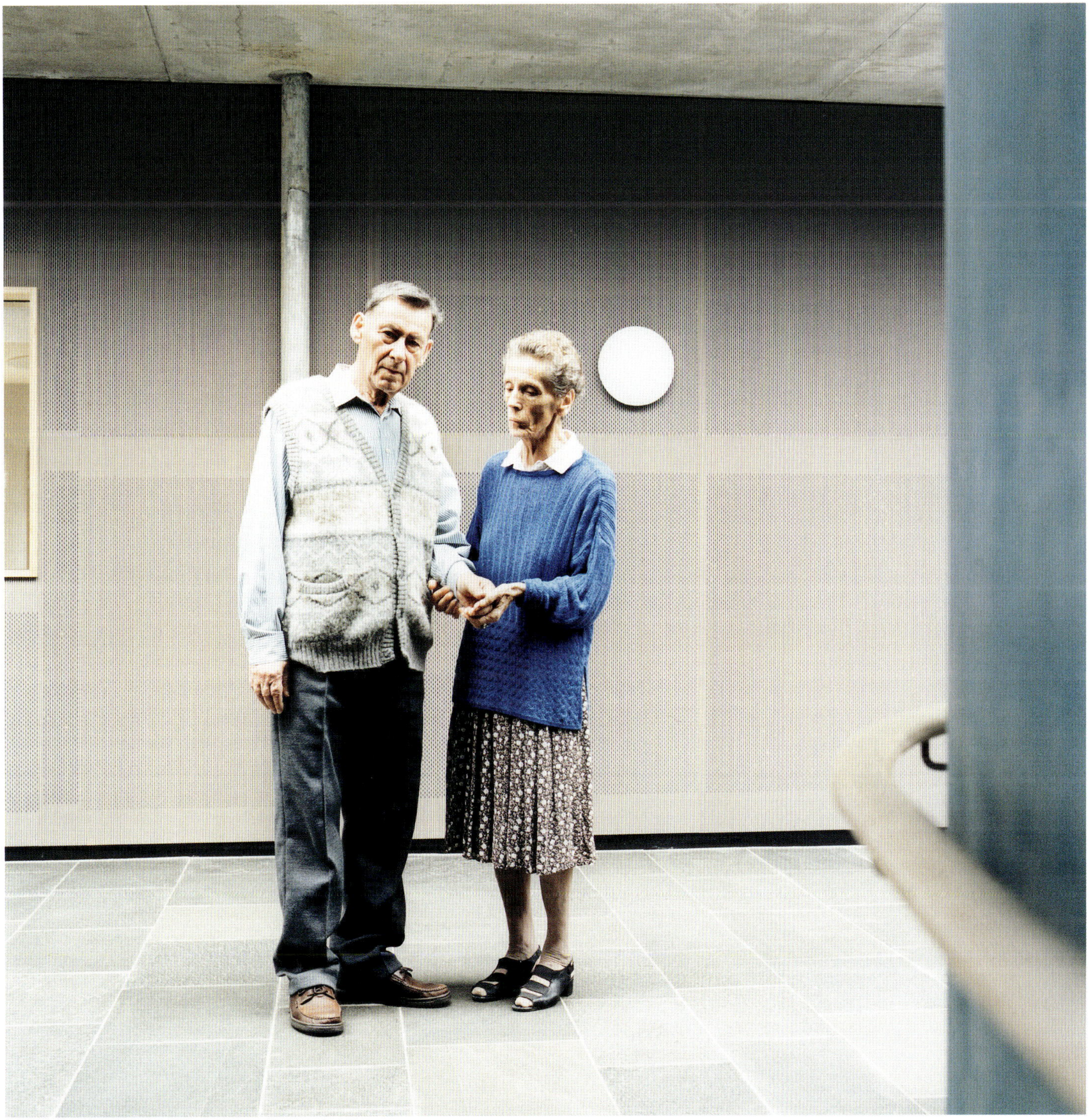

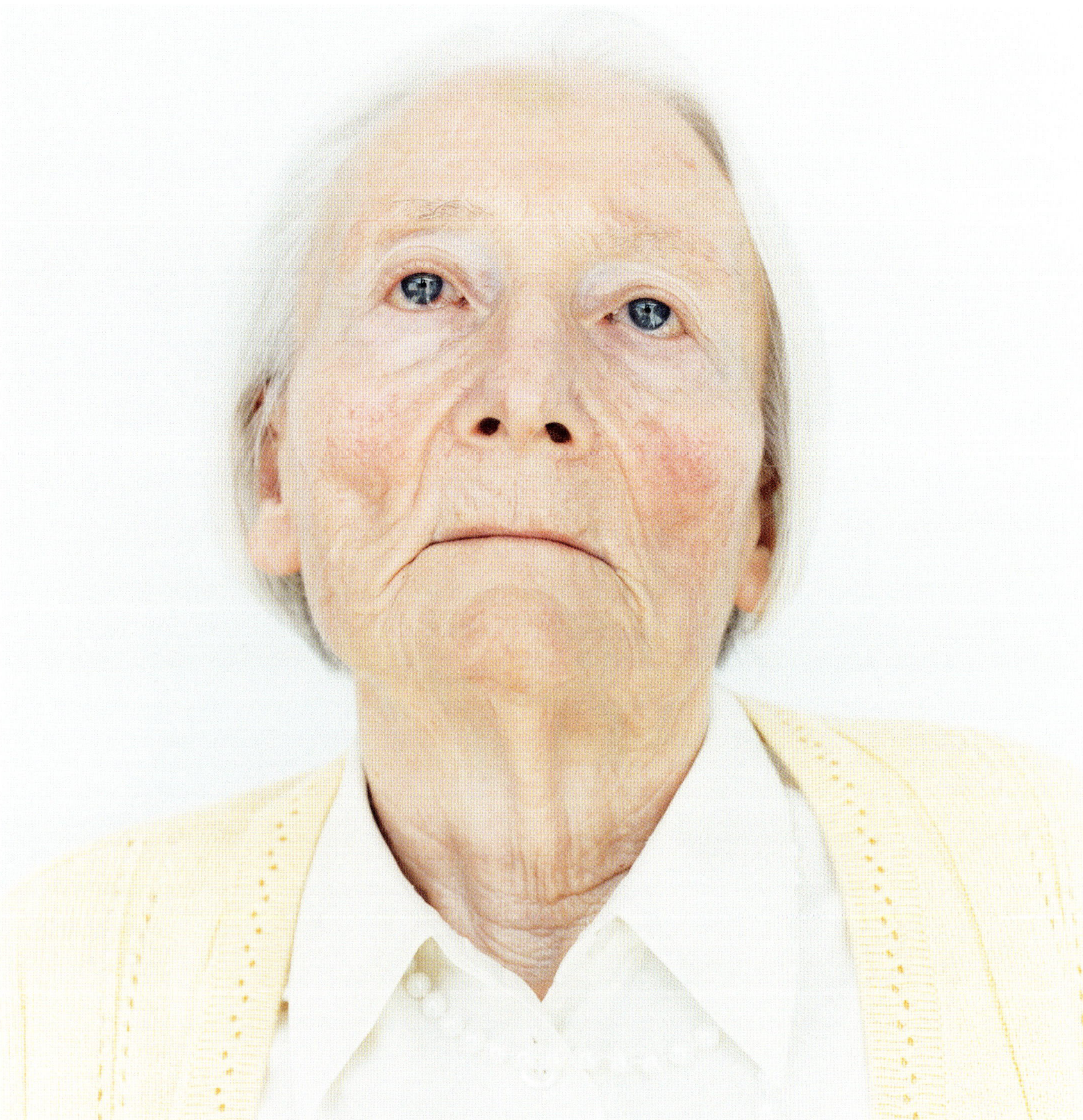

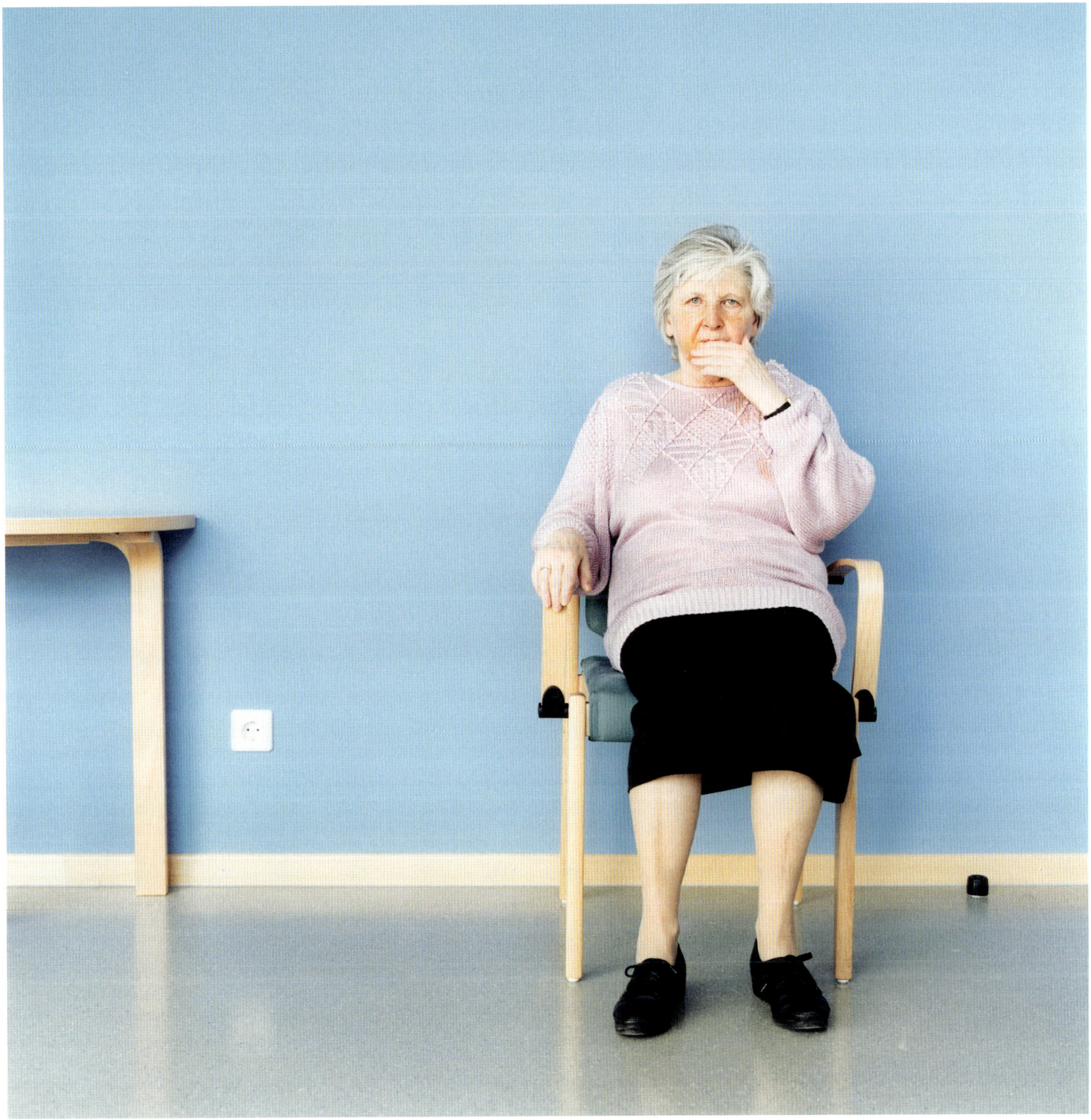

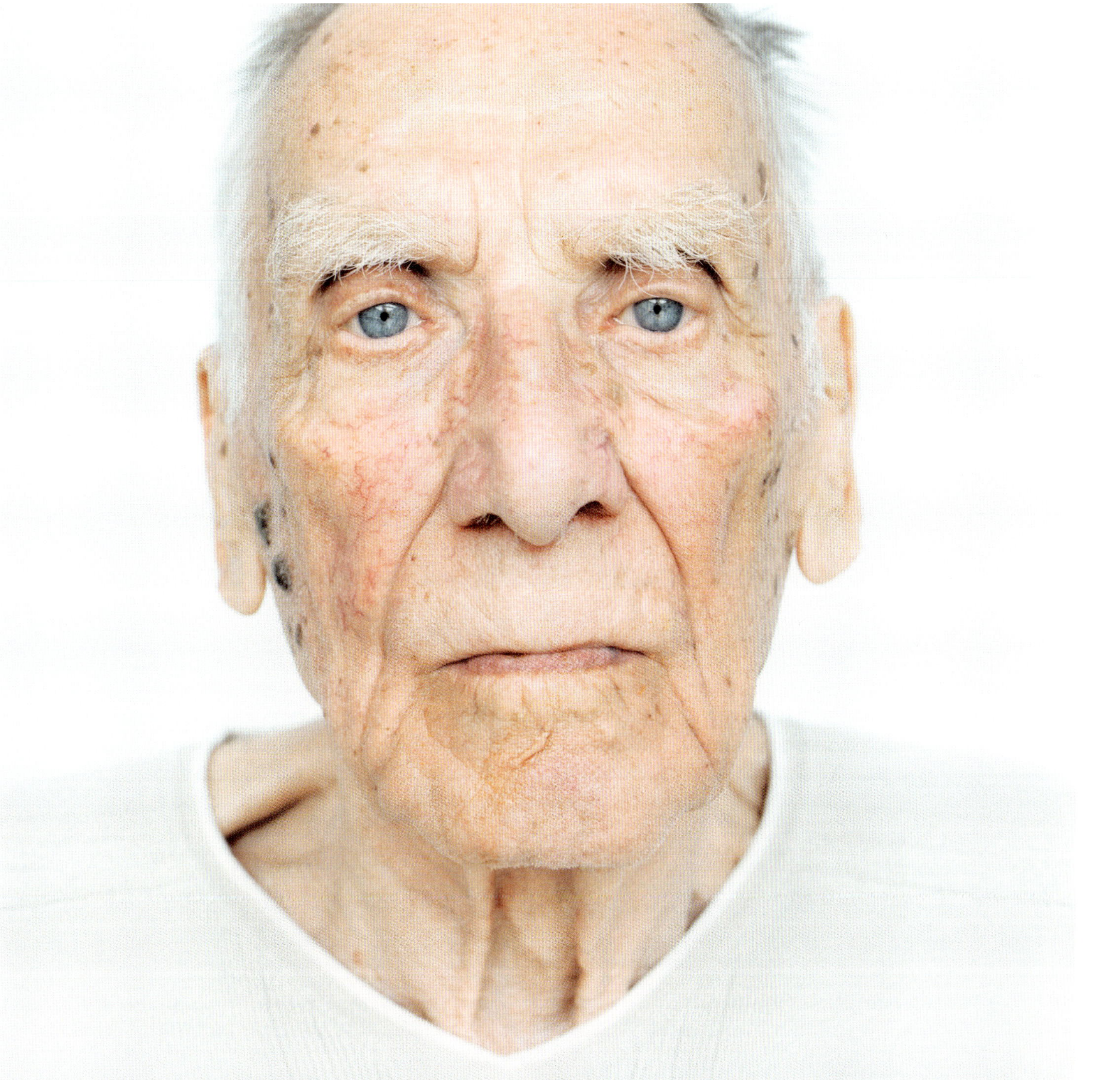

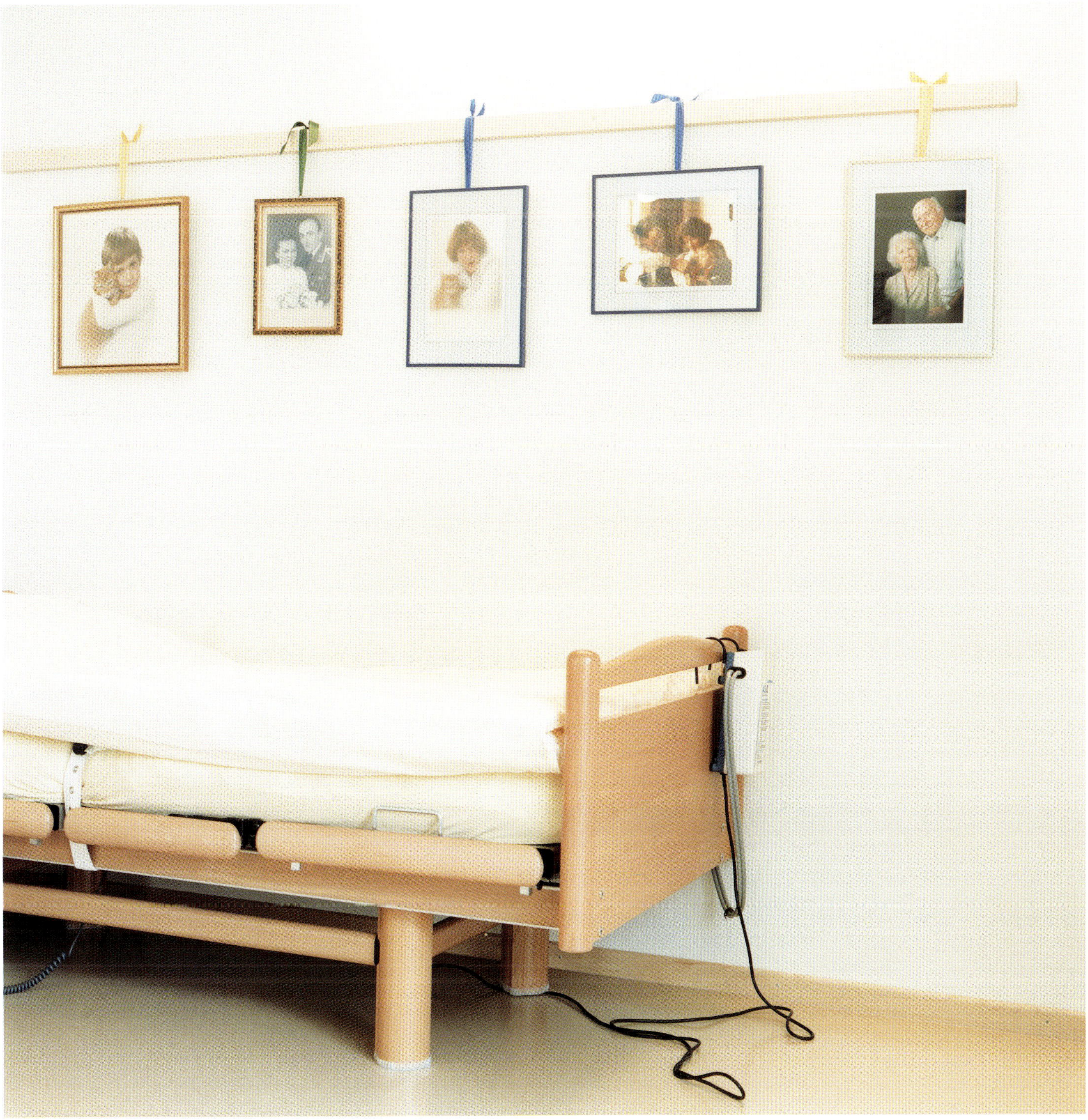

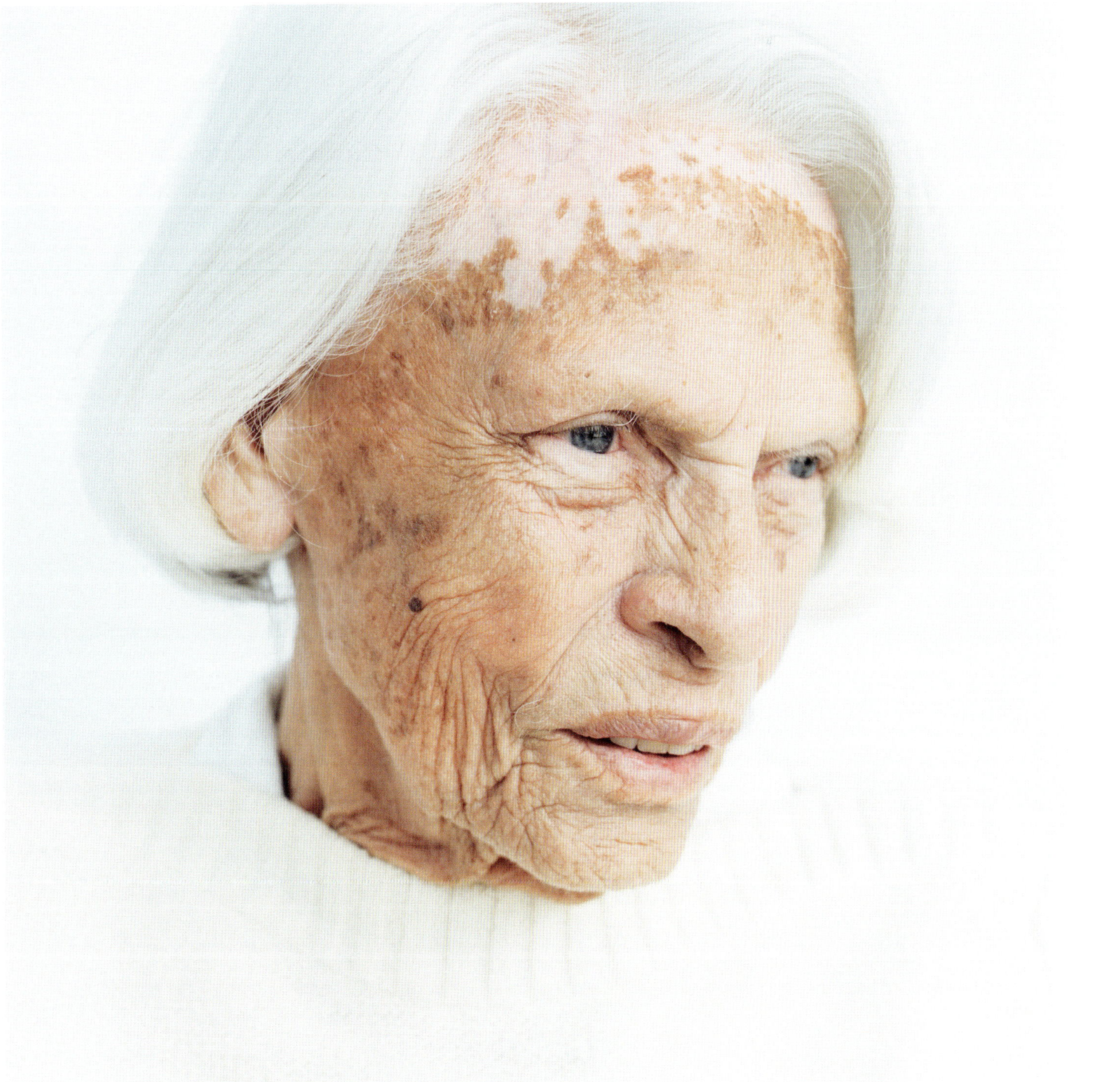

1. "This is a lousy film," says the man to his wife and gets up from his seat. "Let's get out of here." His wife tells him that's impossible and doesn't make any attempt to leave. She's right: the couple is not sitting in a movie theater, but in an airplane. They are on their way to New York City from Amsterdam; underneath them lies the Atlantic, the film is in-flight entertainment, and you can't just get up and leave. The fact that the man nevertheless wants to exit the theater is no joke, but dead serious and a situation encountered almost daily in the life of Alzheimer's victim Willem De Kooning and his wife Elaine.

That was 1983. De Kooning, who was born in Holland and emigrated to the USA as a young man, was one of the most famous American painters of his day. He had his breakthrough in the 1950s, and then suffered from severe alcoholism for decades. He and Elaine separated, got back together, he stopped drinking, stayed with Elaine, and then was diagnosed with suspected Alzheimer's. "Your body's going to last," his wife predicted immediately after receiving the bad news, "but your brain is going to go." She was right on both counts. Although De Kooning was able to rely less and less on his memories and intellectual abilities, he continued to paint. His eyes, his muscles seemed to function independently of his brain. He produced 341 paintings in the space of ten years – pictures showing flowing forms on a white background, in bold elementary colors. They are lighter, more optimistic and cheerful than many of the works he painted in a relatively monotonous vein in his life before Alzheimer's. De Kooning's assistants helped him during this phase, readying his materials and fine-tuning details. But the sweeping brushstrokes, the decisive form-giving power came, despite Alzheimer's, from the artist himself. The distance between him and his memories became wider and wider. But in his pictures, the painter felt at home.

2. Just two decades later, in autumn 2001, Peter Granser boarded a flight to the Netherlands. Along with eleven colleagues from all corners of the world, the young photographer from Stuttgart had been chosen to participate in the "World Press Photo Masterclass", a prestigious international workshop. In Granser's luggage on his trip to Rotterdam were pictures he had taken in Stuttgart's Gradmann Haus, a residential facility for Alzheimer's patients.

Granser knew nothing about De Kooning's late works when he set out to document the everyday life of his protagonists. It is a coincidence that his photographs, with their clarity and radiant brightness, resemble the paintings by the great American artist. Like every year, the "Masterclass" had assigned a specific theme for the young photographers to treat. In 2001 it was the quite fashionable topic of "Identity". Instead of looking at the ways people find their identity – the first kiss, the first pair of jeans from The Gap, freshman year – Granser took an interest in the less attractive end of the spectrum. He focused on Alzheimer's: the assault on the identity, the creeping, inexorable loss of self. At first, he wanted to photograph a community living situation for Alzheimer's patients in Berlin. But then, in order to be able to spend more time on site, he decided instead on a series about the Gradmann Haus close to his home.

Why choose such an awkward theme? The reasons have a lot to do with Granser's curiosity. Unlike many documentary photographers working in German-speaking countries, Granser never went to college. He is an autodidact. At 20 he began working for the local press. He was soon taking photos for national newspapers, and later for magazines. In his spare time he undertook freelance projects that had little to do with his everyday news subjects, but were not conceived in the shadow of an academic taskmaster either. He soon developed his own signature style, with spare, clear-lined pictorial compositions evincing a finely tuned sense of irony. Granser is interested in bizarre, artificial worlds: Austria as a tourists' paradise, New York's Coney Island amusement park, Germans who like to dress up as cowboys for weekend get-togethers where they relive the golden days of the Wild West.

Alzheimer's was a subject to which the photographer did not come wholly unprepared. Before turning his attention to the illness, he had completed work on his *Sun City* project, a series about a retirement colony in the American southwest. In this strange city of spunky senior citizens, he encountered innumerable whimsical details. And then he took wrinkles, cacti, hair dryer hoods and plastic flamingos and compiled them into a basically true and only slightly exaggerated story about the future of aging. In *Sun City* being a senior citizen doesn't mean sitting in a rocking chair on the porch, looking back at the past, gradually taking one's leave of life. Quite the opposite: Granser's picture story is peopled by men and women who without any compromises or sentimentality have radically reinvented themselves in their latter years. His work on Alzheimer's plumbs the other extreme: dependency and vulnerability. As in *Sun City*, however, Granser approaches this world as well with a sense of wonder and not with cynicism.

3. There are not many photo series about Alzheimer's. The reason seems obvious. This is a disease that is first and foremost about language. That's what makes it so frightening: Alzheimer's attacks its victim's cognitive and intellectual faculties, starting with the ability to communicate. Suddenly, there are words that the sufferer can no longer find, write or pronounce; suddenly, he can no longer remember names, they are simply lost, erased from the hard disk. The medical diagnosis is also about language, about simple questions the doctor poses when conducting the so-called SIDAM interview for the diagnosis of dementia ("What year is it?" for example, or: "Who was the first German chancellor after World War II?"). Wrong answers are immediately viewed as symptoms of an incurable illness, which reduces the victim's remaining life expectancy to an average of about eight years. Thus, the moment in which language fails marks the beginning of an ineluctable tragedy, which medication can only halt temporarily. This is why friends and family are so horrified and feel so helpless when everyday conversation suddenly no longer functions. The person they know so well looks exactly the same as ever. But he talks like a stranger.

Alzheimer's can affect anyone, putting even the sharpest intellect into a state of permanent bewilderment. This explains why such a flood of literary texts about this disease has appeared in recent years. Since language is the tool of their trade, writers evidently find this theme especially compelling. The Swiss author Martin Suter made it the basis of his gripping novel, *Small World*. American writer Jonathan Franzen reacted to the dementia and death of his father with a deeply felt essay (*My Father's Brain*) and the tragicomic bestseller *The Corrections*. In a recently published short story by Canadian author Alice Munro (*The Bear Came over the Mountain*), the first sign of Alzheimer's is harmless and comedic – a woman sticks little yellow Post-It notes on her kitchen drawers: here is the silverware, here are the dish towels. But the slow process of leave-taking from this world, recounted by Munro in an almost cool tone, is unstoppable. In her story as well, it is the failure of words that makes this process especially painful.

4. Since words are worth so much in this case, and pictures so little, Peter Granser had to overcome various reservations before he began to take photos at Gradmann Haus. "There is a general problem regarding how photographers are seen by the public," he says. "When people hear the word 'photographer', the first thing that seems to come to mind is: he chases celebrities." Relatively quickly, Granser was able to convince the house management of his careful working methods – assuring them, for example, that he would not be using any spotlights or flashbulbs. But then came the discussions with patients' families. "That was more difficult," he remembers. "What if someone sees what you are doing?" the photographer was asked. Family members were concerned about the reactions of friends, colleagues, acquaintances. Granser visited the facility every day, showed people the photos he had taken, explained his concept, until he finally managed to calm the families' doubts. He recalls one conversation in particular: "A woman told me how much one of my pictures had helped her to accept her husband's struggle with Alzheimer's. Before, she said, she had always clung desperately to the old image she had of him in her mind."

One thing the photographer freely acknowledges is that the facility in which his series is set cannot necessarily be regarded as typical. The Gradmann Haus is a model project. It houses only 24 permanent residents and a day group of 10 to 15 Alzheimer's patients. The architecture is specially designed to fulfill their needs, with lots of daylight, a garden, and long corridors to accommodate the restless movement often associated with the disease. In Stuttgart alone, there are thousands of Alzheimer's sufferers for whom this kind of care would be a blessing. "It is not typical, but it should be typical," says Granser. "I didn't want to show the nursing stations where the patients are simply strapped to their beds. I was interested in showing more simple images, which are still capable of giving us access to this disease, and can convey an impression of the seclusion in which the sufferers live."

In order to open up this access, Granser needed to carefully balance his series. On the one hand, the images put the human being and what he must endure in the foreground. But on the other hand, the photographer shows great respect for the dignity of the patient at all times. Pastel tones shed a flattering light on both men and women; the camera unobtrusively follows their gait, their gestures. The woman smearing her room with feces, the man urinating in the hallway because the concept of "going to the toilet" is no longer familiar: you won't find these scenes in Granser's work. He knew what he didn't want: a continuation of the conventional documentary photography of the 1960s and 1970s, with its almost alienating predilection for dramatizing people's misery, nakedness and weakness. "All good photography is voyeuristic," says photography book publisher Chris Boot, who learned about Granser's project in the "World Press Photo Master Class." "Peter's pictures are not aggressive. Nor are they sentimental."

Color plays a pivotal role in this balancing act. It's like a veil protecting the subjects. Moreover, it helps the photographer to avoid exactly that brand of classic social reporting that always surrounds images of mental illness and dementia with modulated shades of dismal gray. "At some point I realized," says Granser, "that these great role models of black and white photography don't help me with the stories I have to tell." Granser's light colors create distance: "They elevate the pictures above reality," he says. No claim is made to universality. This is just one approach, one perspective, one version of Alzheimer's.

The unwieldy medium format camera gives added reinforcement to this cautious strategy. The photographs are documents of long days, taken during what were sometimes entirely non-eventful visits during which Peter Granser pressed the shutter only two or three times. With his camera and tripod in hand, he moved slowly through the corridors, sometimes letting the residents take him by the hand and lead him. He studied a woman's nightstand: the framed photo of her husband, the "Danone Gran Frutta" yogurt container, the paper tissues from Schlecker drugstore, the comb, the lipstick, the flower arrangement. He photographed movements from a distance: the aimless searching, the hands thrown up in the air. And he avoided a hectic pace and confrontation.

5. Granser's portraits nonetheless manifest a breathtaking immediacy. It is almost impossible to escape the fascination of these faces, to resist getting caught up in contemplating the life stories they represent. Some viewers will have difficulties with the close-ups: after all, there is an unwritten law in modern documentary photography that the relationship between photographer and subject should always be one of equals. We have become accustomed to portraits that overtly express this equality. Portraitists of human peculiarities are quickly deemed condescending today, because the camera has so often been used to expose people, to humiliate them, to categorize them as inferior because of their race, their social background or their mental state. Thus, contemporary documentary portraits usually show individuals brimming with self-confidence, who stare into the lens with such energy and defiance that the viewer is almost taken aback.

The portrait sittings in Gradmann Haus were different. There, only one person knew what was really going on: the photographer (only two of the residents had some idea of what the young man was up to on his way through the hallways and common rooms). The fact that those portrayed are clueless as to what is happening has the effect of neutralizing the artificiality of the photographic act. The men and women don't present themselves to the camera, don't offer up their faces to the photographer's gaze. They are instead driven by the restlessness that Alzheimer's imposes on them. This may very well guarantee authentic portraits. However, critics might note down that it almost constitutes a return to the pictures of the late 19th century, when photographers set out in droves to catalogue the mentally ill.

In order to earnestly pursue this argument, one would have to consistently ignore Peter Granser's images. There are few portrait series by contemporary photographers in which the protagonists are granted so much dignity and so much authority. It is true that, at the moment the shutter closes, Granser knows much more about what is going on than his subjects. He does control a situation that they do not comprehend. But what is the alternative? When journalists and literary figures write about Alzheimer's patients, they are operating on the basis of a much more blatant incongruity. The author exercises the full range of his language skills to express himself, to make his points – whereas the patient by contrast seems to be an inferior being, because he has veered away from the world of language. This is what happened to Auguste D., the patient of Alois Alzheimer. Her wrong answers to simple questions ("What is your husband's name?" – "I think it's Auguste.") mark the beginning of the history of this disease in 1901. The writer Iris Murdoch was subjected to much the same treatment. When Murdoch's husband, John Bayley, told her story in his bestselling memoir *Elegy for Iris*, he had the last word because he had been spared the illness that silenced her. And so the world came to know Murdoch, a philosopher and world-famous author, as a confused old lady who sits listlessly on the couch, only showing signs of glee when the daily episode of the "Teletubbies" comes on. This kind of imbalance is not found in Peter Granser's images. The photographer remains invisible, the protagonists anonymous.

6. We are used to viewing Alzheimer's as a – still – incurable scourge of humanity. We place our hopes in ambitious medical scientists who are

hard at work in laboratories around the world in search of diagnostic methods that could enable the earliest possible detection and treatment. And then there is the more remote goal: the drug that might one day be able to cure the disease. We are sure they will find it someday. So the future may look rosy (if you ask the scientists), but the everyday world of Alzheimer's is still gray.

But there are other voices wanting to be heard. Scientific journalist David Shenk argues that this hypothetical anti-Alzheimer's wonder drug would not really help mankind that much. Shenk wonders if the phase of forgetting isn't just as natural a part of the end of life as learning is part of its beginning. To him, our plan for ridding ourselves of senility sounds like the idea of abolishing winter. In 419 B.C. Aristophanes declared that old men become children once again. At the beginning of the 17th century, Shakespeare had his King Lear bickering with elements of everyday life just like an Alzheimer's patient: "All the skill I have," laments Lear, "remembers not these garments: nor I know not / Where I did lodge last night." If coming to terms with dementia has been part of our culture for thousands of years, if the joys of life are so great only because we know what awaits us in the end: why do we still have such a need to intervene in these processes?

Forgetting, the other side of memory, is what makes us human. For this reason, some observers do not consider the fight against senility to be the most important battle facing mankind. Comparing the disease to AIDS, one becomes more cautious about referring to Alzheimer's as a worldwide epidemic destroying millions of human lives. Unlike AIDS, Alzheimer's is merely a construct – an artificial label used by doctors who at some point decided not to simply accept senile dementia as a natural phenomenon, but instead to define it as a disease and to combat it as such. Unlike AIDS in southern Africa, Alzheimer's is not a catastrophe that threatens to undo our society, but is instead a social challenge. This might be a way to put things in perspective.

These ideas motivate some people to think again about how we view dementia and not to see it as an enemy to be exterminated, but rather as a natural phase of human life. In the USA, scholar Anne Davis Basting, a specialist on aging, is conducting a project called "Time Slips". She organizes discussion rounds with Alzheimer's patients, in which they tell collective stories that are fragmented, non-linear and improvised, out of which theatrical productions are then created. Basting aims to demonstrate in this way how rigid and ultimately artificial our idea is that individuality and creativity completely depend on a perfectly functioning intellect. After all, as we can see from Willem De Kooning's late paintings, there is a form of artistic expression that has no need for clear, rational thinking. Peter Granser's photographs can also be understood in this sense – as arresting attempts at seeing dementia in a new way, without timidity and without panic.

For many people who have watched their loved ones fall victim to Alzheimer's, this concept might seem more than a little strange. Two out of three dementia patients live at home, cared for by family members. Whoever has spent even a single day taking care of someone affected knows about the grim, ugly side of the disease. And now we are asked to accept forgetting as part of life? To view Alzheimer's as a construct, even as a chance for new creativity? That, some might object, is something only theorists could possibly come up with. Those are ideas, it seems, that could only occur to someone whose own mother has never asked him if she hasn't seen him someplace before. Because the process of forgetting is by no means always peaceful and harmonious. Research is increasingly concentrating on the many serious symptoms accompanying the loss of memory. Crippling anxiety can develop, depression, paranoia – and anger and violence directed against family members, even as they are devoting all of their time and energy to caring for the patient. One might criticize that we see nothing of these problems here.

These objections do make sense in the context of the general debate on Alzheimer's. But they are unfounded when it comes to Peter Granser's photo series. Granser does not promise us a comprehensive panorama. His series does not claim to constitute a scientific study. Cautiously, soberly and optimistically, the pictures embark on a dialogue, directing our gaze toward faces and gestures that no one would have otherwise taken the time to observe. Overstatement is not Granser's métier. Once again: this is only a story about the traces that Alzheimer's leaves behind. It's about loss. It's about dignity. And about the radiant contradictions in the human face.

Christoph Ribbat
publishes in the fields of narrative literature, photography and cultural history; he teaches at the University of Bonn, Germany.

The author would like to thank Peter Granser, Gabriele Kreutzner, Ina Schermuly, Jochen Klucken, Alberto Lleo and Chris Boot for their help and advice. David Shenk's outstanding book *The Forgetting: Alzheimer's – Portrait of an Epidemic* (New York, 2001) was indispensable.

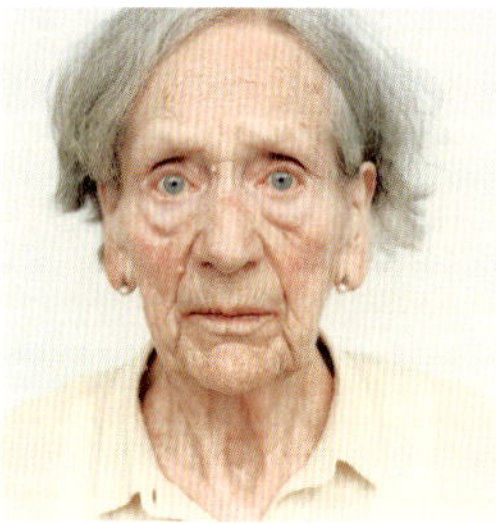
Portrait 1, 2001

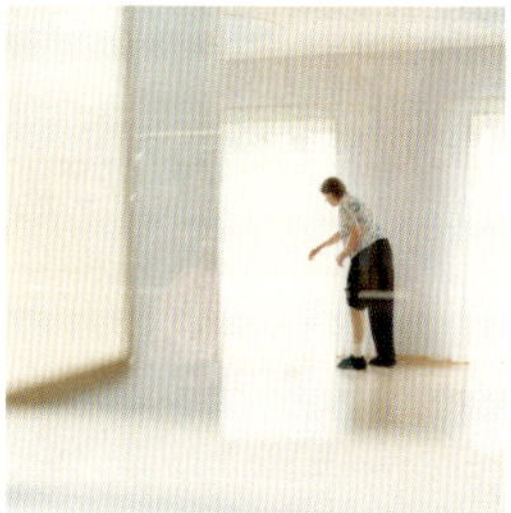
Observation 1, 2001

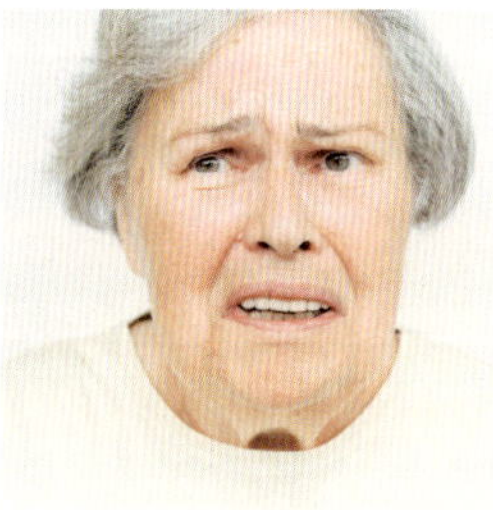
Portrait 2, 2001

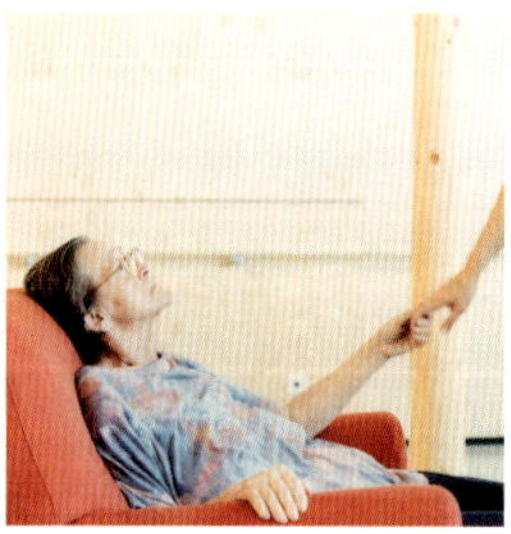
Observation 2, 2001

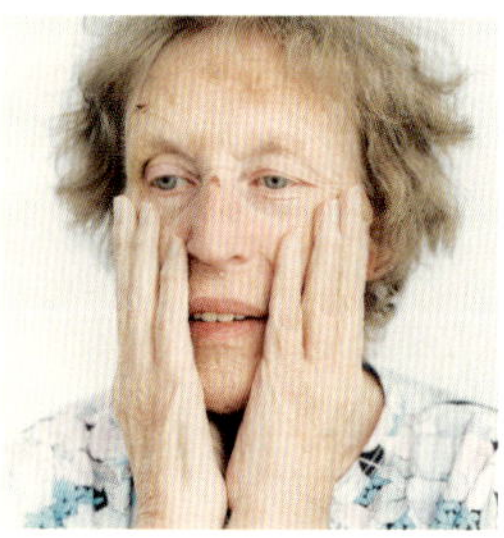
Portrait 3, 2001

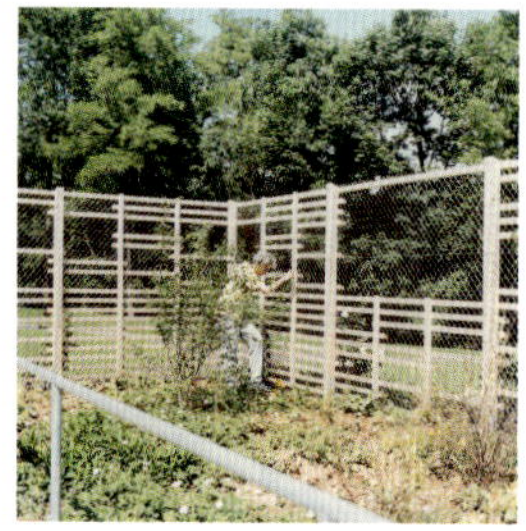
Observation 3, 2001

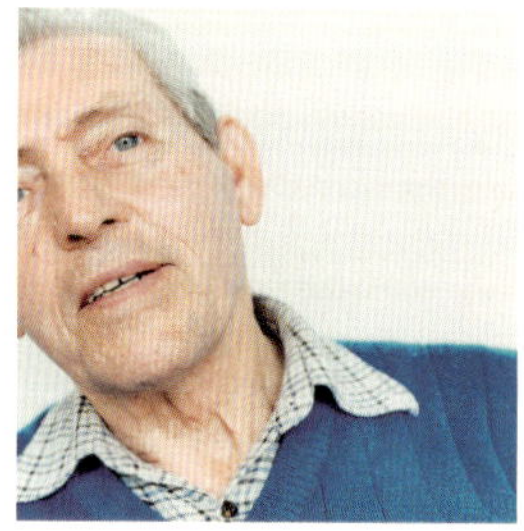
Portrait 4, 2004

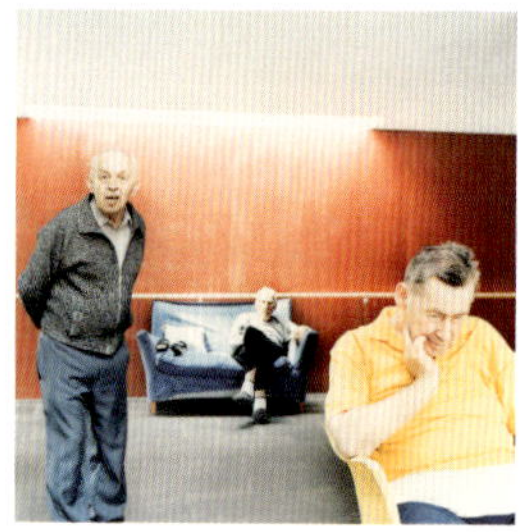
Observation 4, 2004

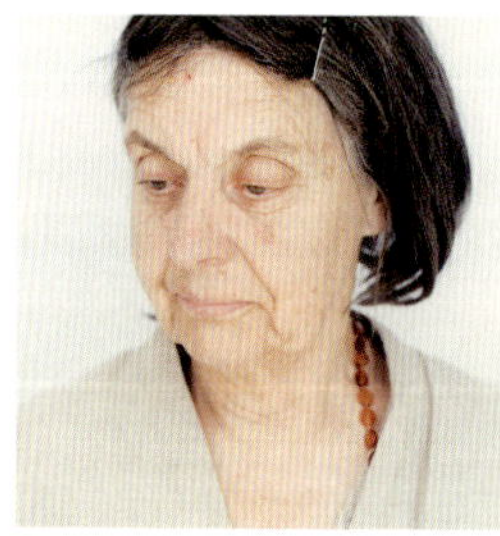
Portrait 5, 2004

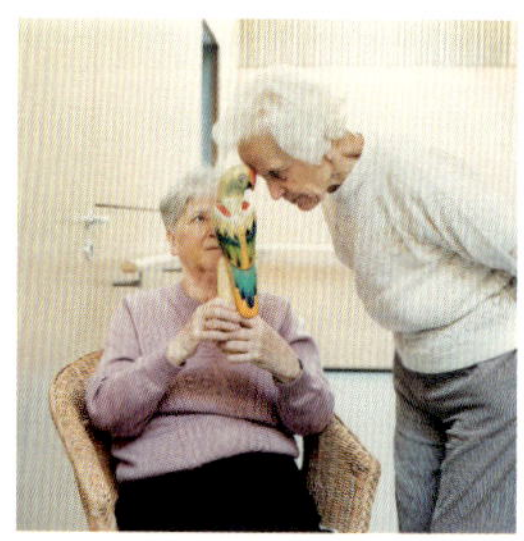
Observation 5, 2001

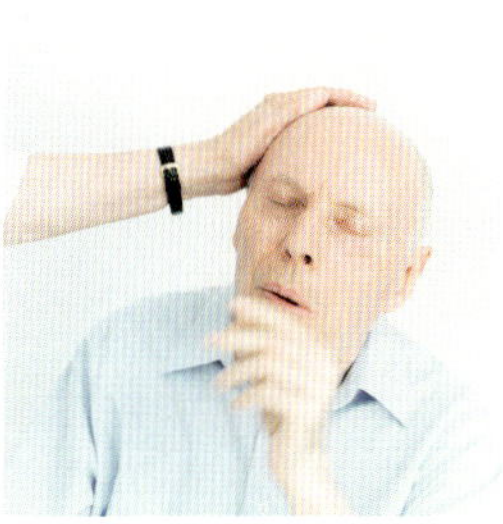

Portrait 6, 2001

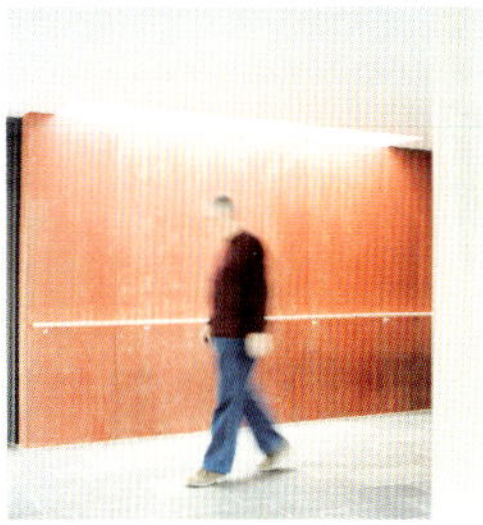

Observation 6, 2001

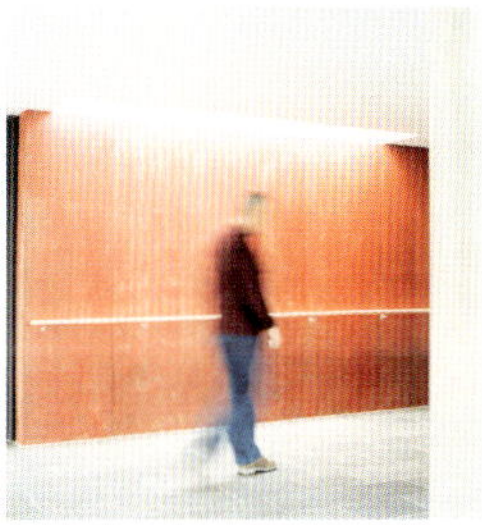

Observation 7, 2001

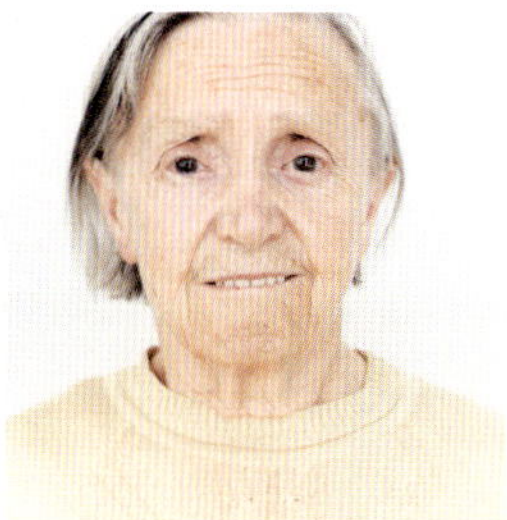

Portrait 7, 2004

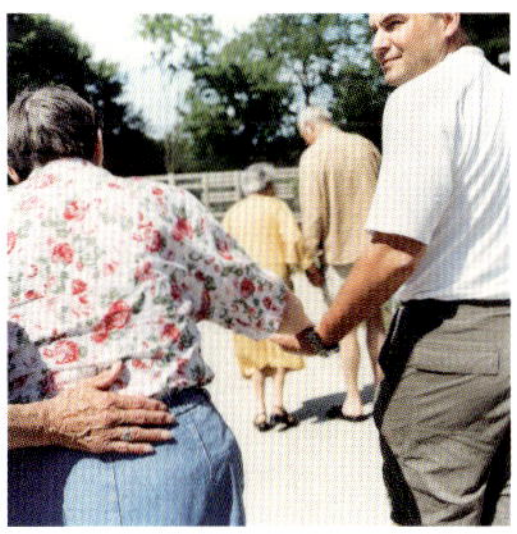

Observation 8, 2001

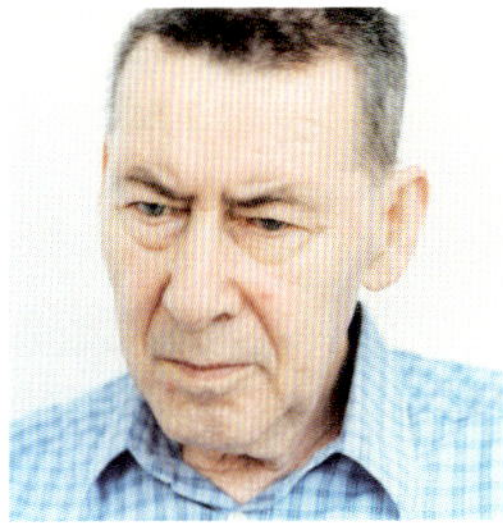

Portrait 8, 2001

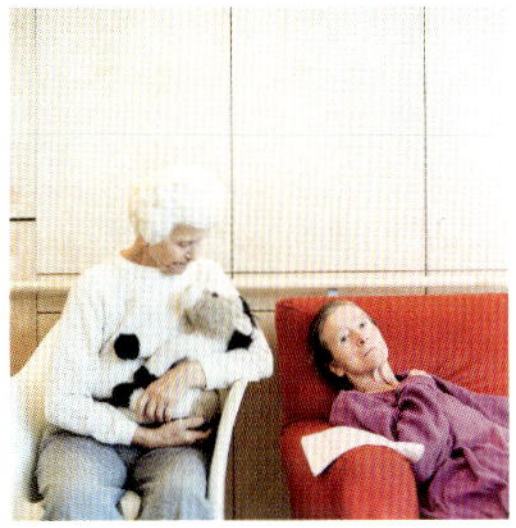

Observation 9, 2001

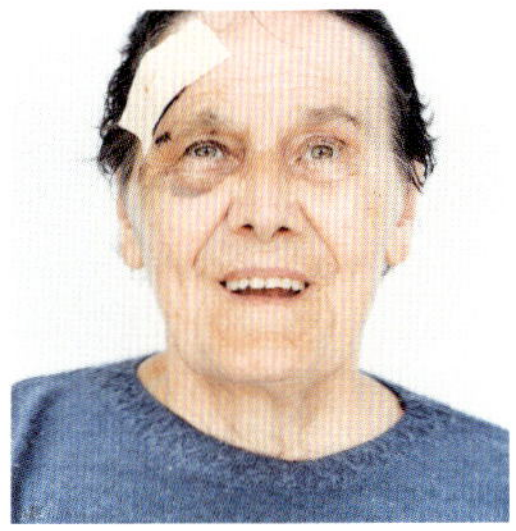

Portrait 9, 2004

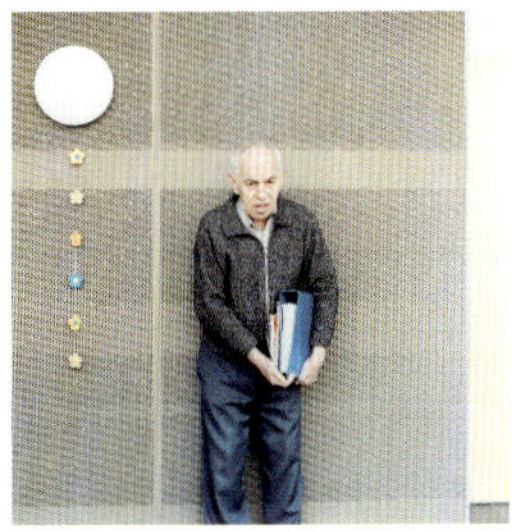

Observation 10, 2004

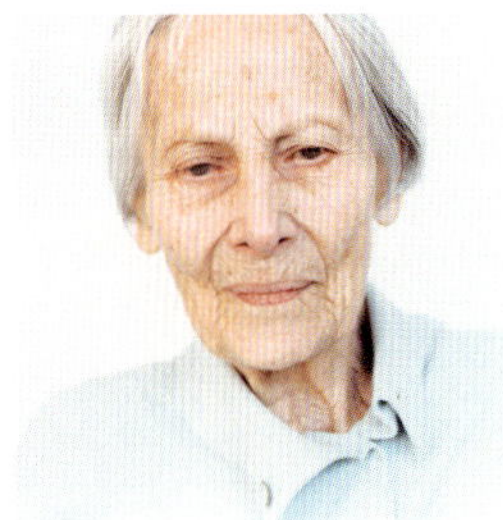

Portrait 10, 2004

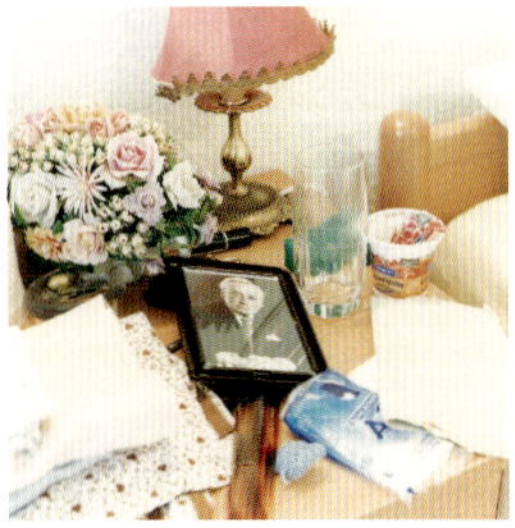

Observation 11, 2001

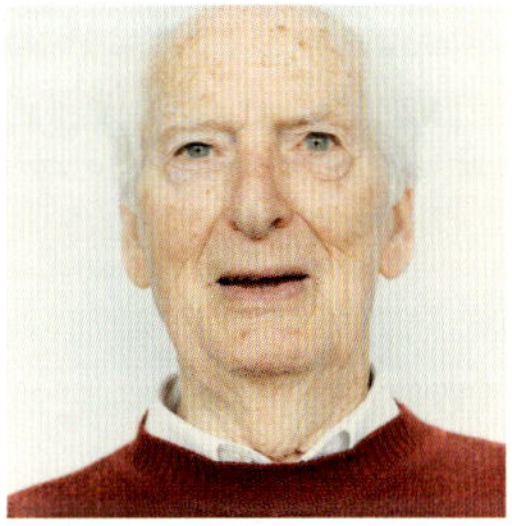

Portrait 11, 2004

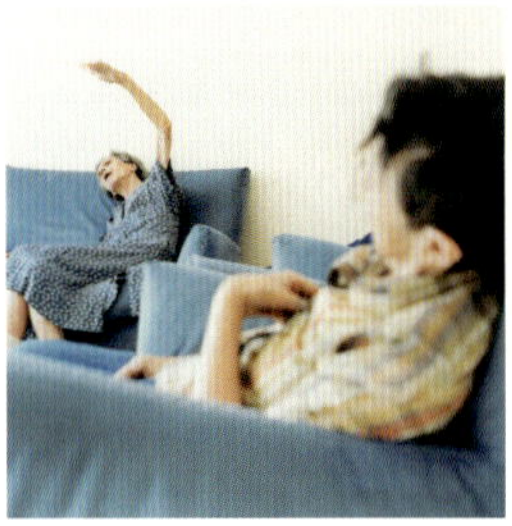

Observation 12, 2001

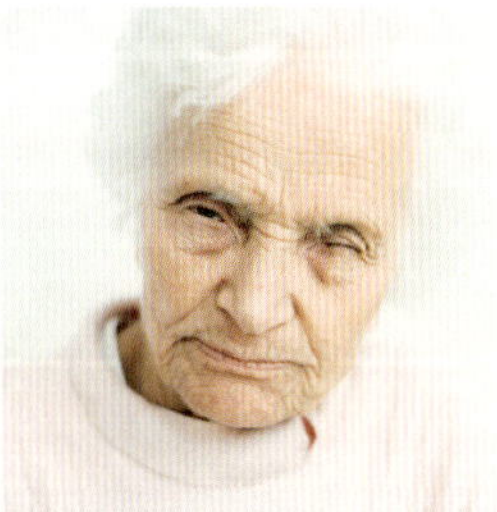

Portrait 12, 2001

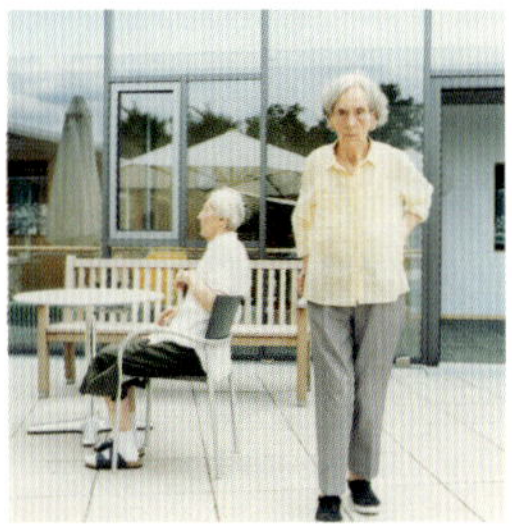

Observation 13, 2001

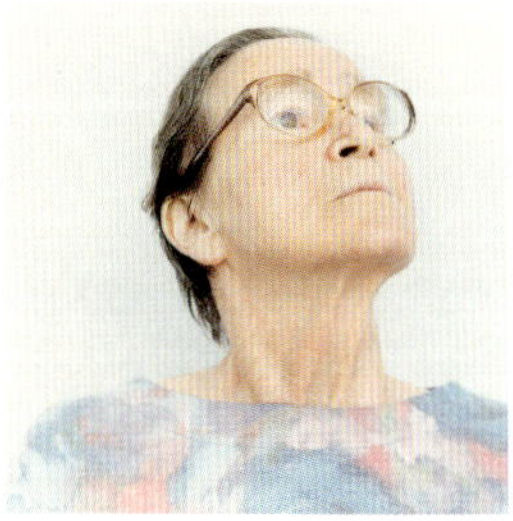

Portrait 13, 2001

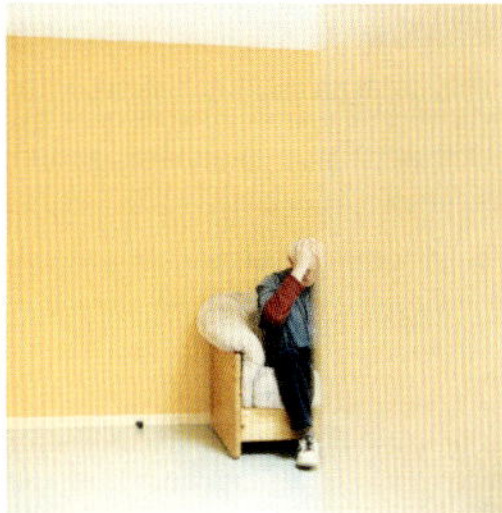

Observation 14, 2001

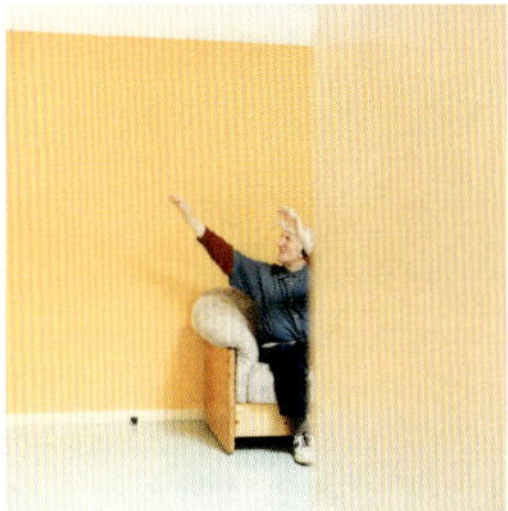

Observation 15, 2001

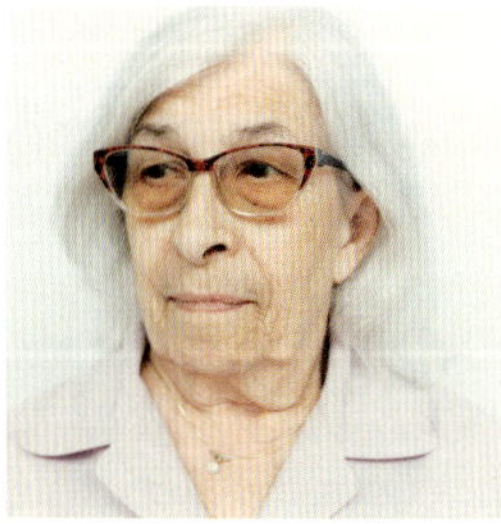

Portrait 14, 2004

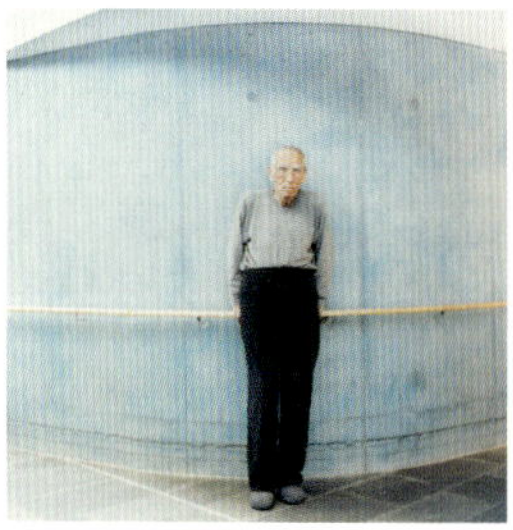

Observation 16, 2004

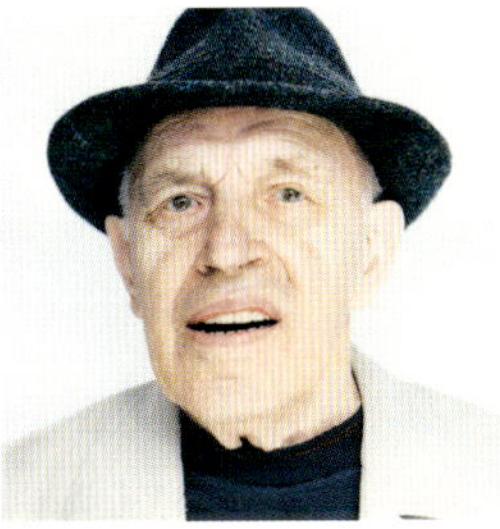

Portrait 15, 2004

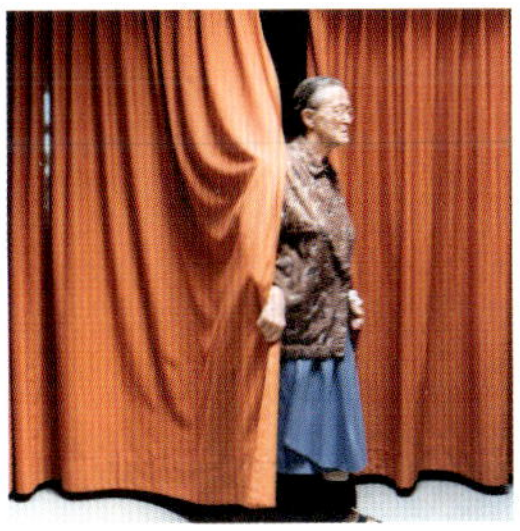

Observation 17, 2001

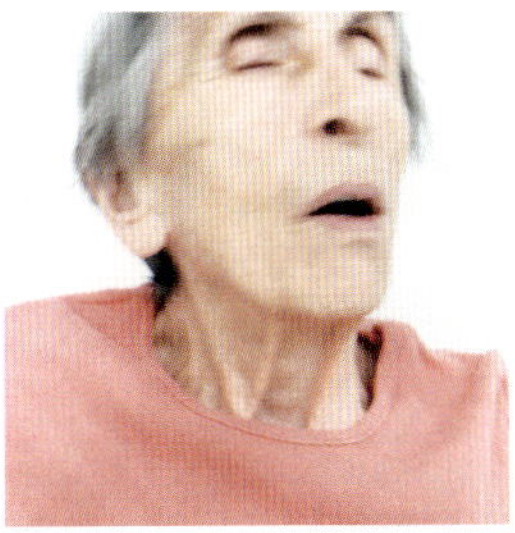

Portrait 16, 2001

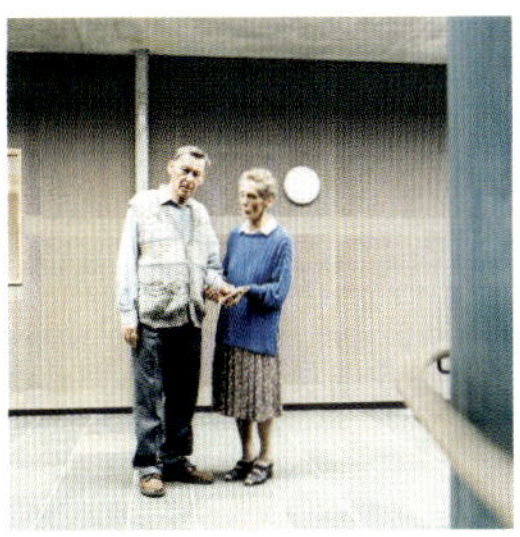

Observation 18, 2001

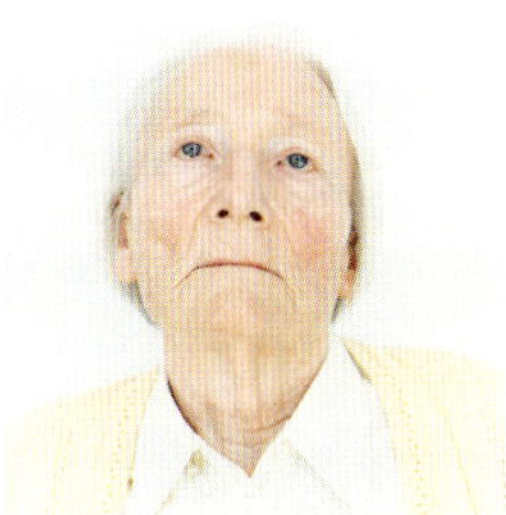

Portrait 17, 2004

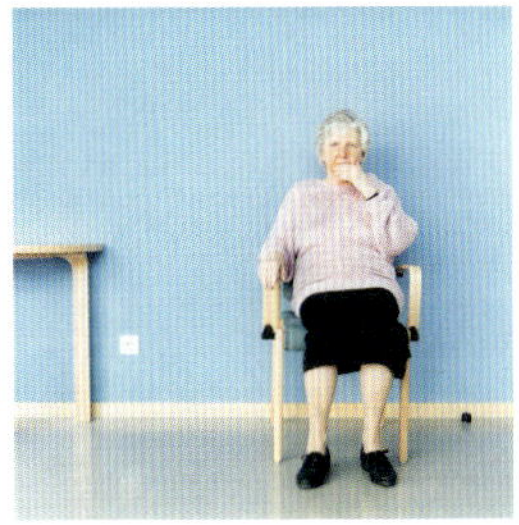

Observation 19, 2001

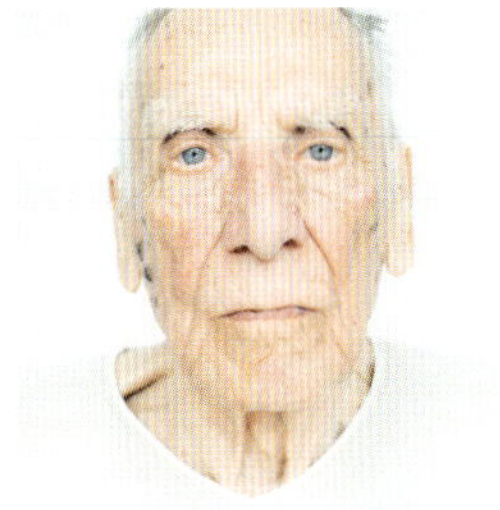

Portrait 18, 2004

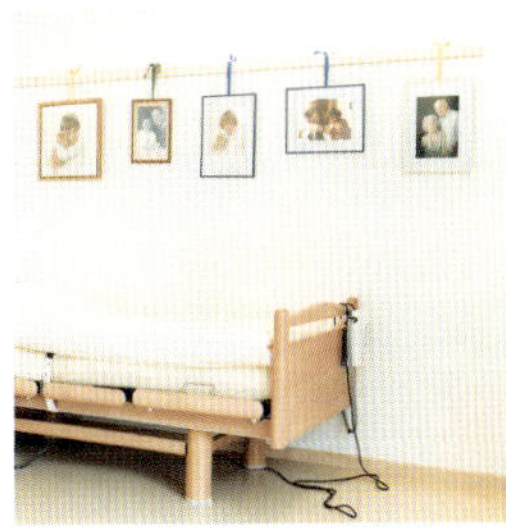

Observation 20, 2001

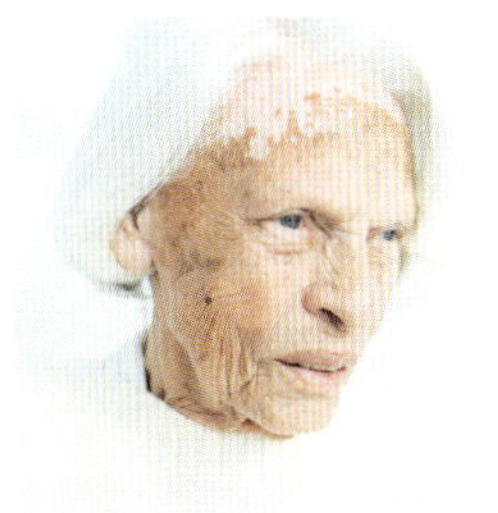

Portrait 19, 2001

Schon immer haben Stiftungen besondere Themen der Zeit aufgegriffen und neue Wege gesucht, bevor Staat und Gesellschaft dafür Steuermittel einsetzen können. Das Ehepaar Gradmann aus Ostfildern bei Stuttgart, vermögend geworden durch den Aufbau einer bedeutenden Versicherungsagentur, beschloss, sein Vermögen dazu einzusetzen, hilfebedürftige ältere Menschen insbesondere durch Schaffung von Wohnraum zu unterstützen. Nach ihrem Tod im Jahre 1991 wurde die Erich und Liselotte Gradmann-Stiftung mit Sitz in Stuttgart ins Leben gerufen.

Die Stiftung baut und fördert seither innovative Projekte im Bereich der Altenhilfe, die ohne dieses Engagement nicht entstehen würden. Zwei Betreute Wohnanlagen mit Stadtteiltreffpunkt, ein Pflegeheim in Ostfildern und das Gradmann Haus in Stuttgart-Kaltental, ein Zentrum für Demenzkranke mit Betreutem Wohnen, zeugen davon. Bei den Projekten wird jeweils der aktuelle Forschungsstand zum Gebäudedesign für Ältere umgesetzt, die enge Kooperation mit der Universität Stuttgart sichert eine kritische Begleitung und Auswertung der „gebauten Experimente".

Die Stiftung erkannte bald, dass im Bereich der Altenhilfe nicht der Mangel an Wohnraum, sondern die mangelnde Anpassung an neue Herausforderungen besondere Probleme aufwirft. Dazu gehört vor allem auch die dramatisch wachsende Zahl von Menschen, die an Altersdemenz leiden. In der Folge verlagerte sich der Aktivitätenschwerpunkt der Stiftung vom Gebäudedesign für Ältere zum Wissenstransfer im Bereich Demenz.

Die als Tochter der Gradmann-Stiftung im Jahr 2002 gegründete Demenz Support Stuttgart – Zentrum für Informationstransfer – forscht, berät, informiert und qualifiziert seither mit dem Ziel, die Lebensqualität von Menschen mit Demenz zu verbessern. Dabei stehen die Pflege und Betreuung, aber auch die Wohnsituation und die bauliche Anpassung an die spezifischen Bedürfnisse im Mittelpunkt. Wichtiges Lern- und Erfahrungsfeld ist dabei das Gradmann Haus in Stuttgart-Kaltental, das von der Evangelischen Gesellschaft Stuttgart in Zusammenarbeit mit der Alzheimer Gesellschaft Baden-Württemberg betrieben wird.

Die 2001 in Betrieb genommene Einrichtung ist bundesweit das erste Zentrum für Demenzkranke, bei dem eine für Menschen mit Demenz idealtypische Architektur umgesetzt ist. Es wurde inzwischen mehrfach dafür ausgezeichnet. Auch die Konzeption für Pflege und Betreuung greift die neuesten Entwicklungen in Europa auf. Es geht darum, die bisher dominierende institutionell geprägte Versorgung abzulösen durch ein Konzept der „Betreuten Wohngemeinschaft", bei dem der Tagesablauf und die Umgebung am „Leben wie Zuhause" orientiert sind.

Es darf aufgestanden werden, wann man es gewohnt ist. Die Betreuenden sind vertraut mit der Biographie der Bewohner und wissen, dass sie einen ehemaligen Ministerialbeamten oder eine Bibliothekarin als Gegenüber haben, wenn sie mit den Bewohnern reden. In den Zimmern finden sich die eigenen Möbel und auf der Kommode stehen die Fotos der Enkel, wie immer schon. Gegessen wird gemeinsam im Essbereich mit offener Küche, der im Mittelpunkt der Wohngemeinschaft liegt, und in dem immer etwas los ist.

Unruhige Naturen umrunden das Atrium oder spazieren in der verglasten Wandelhalle auf und ab, in der sie immer jemanden finden, mit dem sie ein Schwätzchen halten können. Dort treffen sie auch auf die Gäste der Tagespflege und gehen manchmal einfach mit in den sonnendurchfluteten Aufenthaltsraum, in dem oft gesungen und erzählt wird. Vom Garten aus kann man zu den Betreuten Altenwohnungen hinaufschauen, wo im Idealfall der Ehepartner in einer der barrierefrei gebauten Wohnungen lebt, um seinem kranken Angehörigen möglichst nahe zu sein.

Die Portraits in diesem Band zeigen Menschen mit schweren Ausprägungen von Demenz, die im Gradmann Haus leben oder gelebt haben. Die Bilder spiegeln die Verunsicherung wider, die der Verlust des Gedächtnisses mit sich bringt. Sie sind aber auch – für den, der sehen kann – ein Zeugnis dafür, dass es gelingen kann, auch im oft negativ belegten Kontext eines Pflegeheims eine Umgebung zu schaffen, die Sicherheit und Vertrautheit bietet und die Persönlichkeit des Einzelnen stützt, sodass auch Momente der Heiterkeit und Gelassenheit Raum haben.

Wir sind dem jungen Fotografen Peter Granser dankbar für seinen sensiblen, nie stigmatisierenden, aber auch nie kaschierenden Blick auf die besondere Realität dieser Menschen.

Sibylle Heeg
für die Stiftung, verantwortlich für die Konzeption und bauliche Realisierung des Gradmann Hauses Stuttgart-Kaltental

A Project of the Erich and Liselotte Gradmann Foundation

Foundations have always shown a willingness to take up the pressing issues of their day and find new approaches to them, before the state and society can begin directing tax money toward solutions. The Gradmanns of Ostfildern near Stuttgart, founders of a prominent insurance agency, are a good example. They resolved to devote the wealth they had accumulated during their lifetime to supporting elderly people in need of assistance, especially by providing them with suitable living space. After Mrs. Gradmann's death in 1991, the Erich and Liselotte Gradmann Foundation was established in Stuttgart.

The foundation builds and funds innovative elderly assistance projects that would not be possible without its help. Two assisted living facilities with a neighborhood meeting place, a nursing home in Ostfildern, and the Gradmann Haus in Stuttgart-Kaltental, an assisted living center for dementia sufferers, are testaments to the foundation's work and commitment. Each project applies the current state of knowledge with regard to what constitutes appropriate building design for the elderly, while close cooperation with the University of Stuttgart ensures critical supervision and evaluation of the "constructed experiments".

As the foundation soon realized, the true problem facing us today in the field of elderly assistance is not a lack of living space, but rather the lack of residences that meet current challenges. These include above all the dramatically growing number of people suffering from senile dementia. Consequently, the focus of the foundation's activities soon shifted from building for the elderly to knowledge transfer in the field of dementia.

A subsidiary of the Gradmann Foundation was established in 2002: Demenz Support Stuttgart – Center for Information Transfer. The center conducts research and provides information, consulting and training with the aim of improving the quality of life of people with dementia. Care and assistance for dementia sufferers are provided and structural changes are made to their living situation as required to adapt it to their own specific needs. Important lessons are learned and experience gathered at the Gradmann Haus in Stuttgart-Kaltental, which is run by the Protestant Association of Stuttgart in cooperation with the Alzheimer's Society of Baden-Württemberg.

This facility, which opened its doors in 2001, is Germany's first center for dementia patients in which the architecture is ideally tailored to their needs; the success of the concept has since been recognized with several awards. The care and assistance approach at the facility also incorporates the latest developments in Europe. The goal is to replace the institutional care model that has predominated until now with a concept known as the "assisted community", in which the daily routine and the surroundings are designed to approximate "living at home".

People can get up in the morning at whatever time they're used to. The caregivers know the biography of each resident and realize, for example, that they are speaking not just to a dementia patient, but to a former ministry official or librarian. Residents can equip their rooms with furniture from home, and set photos of the grandchildren on the dresser, just where they have always stood. Meals are eaten in a common dining area with open kitchen, which is at the center of the living community and where there is always something going on.

Restless souls can walk around the atrium or stroll up and down the glassed-in promenade, where they will always find someone to chat with. They also meet up with day guests there and sometimes simply join them in the sunlit common room, where there is often singing and storytelling to be enjoyed. From the garden one can look up to the windows of the assisted living quarters, where ideally a spouse might be residing in a barrier-free apartment in order to be as close as possible to his loved one.

The portraits in this volume show people with severe cases of dementia who live or have lived at the Gradmann Haus. These images reflect the anxiousness and uncertainty that accompanies the loss of one's memory. However, for those who can see clearly, they also testify to the ability to create a nursing home where, instead of the usual negative associations, the atmosphere offers the inhabitants a comfortable feeling of security and familiarity. Here, the personality of each individual is given space to unfold, making way for moments of calm and good cheer.

We would like to thank the young photographer Peter Granser for his sensitive, unflinching but never stigmatizing view of the special reality in which these people live.

Sibylle Heeg
on behalf of the Foundation, responsible for the conception and building
of the Gradmann Haus in Stuttgart-Kaltental

PETER GRANSER

1971	geboren in Hannover, österreichischer Staatsbürger / born in Hannover, Germany, Austrian citizen
1991	erster Kontakt zur Fotografie / first contact with photography
2001	Stipendium / Scholarship World Press Photo Joop Swart Masterclass, Rotterdam, Niederlande / Netherlands
2003	Berufung in die Deutsche Fotografische Akademie / Appointment at the DFA (German Photographic Academy)
2004	Aufnahme in die Künstlergruppe POC-Project / Joins the artist group POC-Project (www.pocproject.com)

Preise und Stipendien / Awards and Grants (ab / from 2001)

2001	Internationaler Preis für jungen Bildjournalismus / International Award for young Photo-Journalists (Anerkennung / selection)
2002	World Press Photo Awards (3. Preis / 3rd prize) Discovery Award, Rencontres d´Arles, Frankreich / France Deutscher Sozialpreis / German Social Award
2003	Europäischer Architektur Fotopreis / European Architecture Photography Award (Anerkennung / selection) Stuttgarter Fotobuchpreis / German Photography Book Award Internationaler Preis für jungen Bildjournalismus / International Award for young Photo-Journalists (Anerkennung / selection) UMBO Fotopreis / Photography Award (Finalist / finalist)
2004	Saar-Förderpreis für junge Kunst / Saar Award for young Art (Finalist / finalist) Oskar-Barnack-Preis /Oskar Barnack Award
2005	Hansel-Mieth-Preis / Hansel Mieth Award (Anerkennungen / selections) World Press Photo Award (ehrenvolle Erwähnung / honorable mention)

Einzelausstellungen / Solo exhibitions (ab / from 2001)

2001	Galerie 11, Hamburg, Germany Galerie photonet, Wiesbaden, Germany
2002	Fondazione Marangoni, Florenz / Florence, Italien / Italy Galerie 14-1, Stuttgart, Germany
2003	Neue Börse, Frankfurt, Germany Photo España , Madrid, Spanien / Spain Galerie photonet, Wiesbaden, Germany
2004	Galerie Kamel Mennour, Paris, Frankreich / France Galerie 14-1, Stuttgart, Germany Galerie 11, Hamburg, Germany
2005	Belfast Exposed, Nordirland / Northern Ireland Estivales Photographiques du Trégor, L'Imagerie, Lannion, Frankreich / France Internationale Fototage / International Photofestival Mannheim und /and Ludwigshafen, Germany Sala El Águila, Consejería de Cultura y Deportes de la Comunidad de Madrid, Spanien / Spain Galerie 14-1, Stuttgart, Germany Centre culturel Les Chiroux, Liège, Belgien / Belgium

Gruppenausstellungen / Group exhibitions (ab / from 2001)

2001 Internationaler Preis für jungen Bildjournalismus, Wanderausstellung / International Award for young Photo-Journalists, Touring exhibition, Germany
Netherlands-Foto-Institut (NFI), Rotterdam, Niederlande / Netherlands
2002 Oude Kerk, Amsterdam, Niederlande / Netherlands
Visual Gallery of Photokina, Köln / Cologne, Germany
Galerie Maximilian Krips, Köln / Cologne, Germany
World Press Photo Wanderausstellung weltweit / Touring exhibition worldwide
Galerie 14-1, Stuttgart, Germany
Galerie Lichtblick, Köln / Cologne, Germany
2003 Internationaler Preis für jungen Bildjournalismus, Wanderausstellung / International Award for young Photo-Journalists, Touring exhibition, Germany
Bundeskunsthalle, Bonn und /and Stadtmuseum Oldenburg, Germany
Städtische Galerie Lippstadt, Germany
Galerie l'Usine, Brüssel / Brussels, Belgien / Belgium
2004 Galerieschiff Frankfurt und / and Kulturbahnhof Eller, Düsseldorf, Germany
KAZ Kunstbahnhof, Kassel, Germany
Saarland Museum, Saarbrücken; TUFA, Trier;
Kunstverein Ludwigshafen, Germany
Dialekt Festival, Stuttgart, Germany
Forum für Fotografie, Köln / Cologne, Germany
Rencontres d´Arles, Frankreich / France
2005 Museum für Photographie, Burghausen, Germany
Galerie Altes Rathaus Musberg, Germany

Repräsentiert durch / Represented by

Galerie Kamel Mennour, Paris, Frankreich / France
Galerie 14-1, Stuttgart, Germany

Sammlungen / Collections

Fotomuseum Winterthur, Schweiz / Switzerland
Staatsgalerie Stuttgart, Grafische Sammlung / Graphic Collection, Germany
LBBW Kunstsammlung, Stuttgart, Germany
Regierungspräsidium / House of Regional Council Stuttgart, Germany
Private Sammler / Private collectors

Bücher / Books

2003 „Sun City" Benteli Verlag, Bern, Schweiz / Switzerland
2005 „Alzheimer" – Kehrer Verlag, Heidelberg, Germany

Mein besonderer Dank gilt den Bewohnern des Gradmann Hauses. Ebenso möchte ich mich für das Vertrauen, die Kooperation und die Unterstützung bei den Angehörigen der Kranken, Herrn Schwarz von der Alzheimer Beratung, Frau Markert, Herrn Peters und den Mitarbeitern des Gradmann Hauses bedanken.

Ich danke allen Förderern des Buches, insbesondere der Gradmann-Stiftung, der Robert Bosch Stiftung, dem Kompetenznetz Demenzen, Ruth Eichhorn von Geo, Prolab Stuttgart, Jörg Walz von der Galerie 14-1, Stuttgart, Kamel Mennour von der Galerie Mennour, Paris, La Fábrica, Madrid, der World Press Foundation, Amsterdam, und dem Kehrer Verlag Heidelberg.

Nicht zu vergessen meiner geliebten Beatrice für ihre Unterstützung, Beratung und ihr Verständnis, wenn ich mal wieder lange Tage beim Fotografieren verbracht habe.

Peter Granser

My special thanks go to the inhabitants of Gradmann House. Further I would like to express my thanks for the trust, the co-operation and the support that I received from the patients' relatives, from Mr. Schwarz of Alzheimer Counseling, Mrs. Markert, Mr. Peters and the staff of Gradmann Haus.

Many thanks to all the supporters of this book; to the Gradmann Foundation, the Robert Bosch Foundation, the Competence Network Dementia, to Ruth Eichhorn from Geo Magazine, to Prolab Stuttgart, to Jörg Walz from Galerie 14-1, Stuttgart, to Kamel Mennour from Galerie Mennour, Paris, to La Fábrica, Madrid, to the World Press Foundation, Amsterdam, and to Kehrer Verlag Heidelberg.

Not to forget, very special thanks to my beloved Beatrice, for her support, her advice and her understanding, whenever I spent long days taking photographs and forgetting time.

Peter Granser

Texte / Texts:
Fritz A. Henn, Christoph Ribbat, Sibylle Heeg

Redaktion / Copy Editing:
Barbara Karpf

Übersetzung / Translation:
Jennifer Taylor-Gaida

Verlagslektorat / Proofreading:
Andrea Hammer

Gestaltung und Herstellung / Design and production:
Kehrer Design Heidelberg

www.kehrerverlag.com
www.granser.de / www.pocproject.com
www.demenz-support.de
www.kompetenznetz-demenzen.de

Kehrer Verlag Heidelberg
ISBN 3-936636-34-6

Bibliografische Information Der Deutschen Bibliothek
Die Deutsche Bibliothek verzeichnet diese Publikation in der Deutschen Nationalbibliografie; detaillierte bibliografische Daten sind im Internet über http://dnb.ddb.de abrufbar.

Bibliographic information published by Die Deutsche Bibliothek
Die Deutsche Bibliothek lists this publication in the Deutsche Nationalbibliografie; detailed bibliographic data are available in the Internet at http://dnb.ddb.de.

Mit freundlicher Unterstützung von

TRUMPF Trumpf GmbH+Co. AG, Ditzingen

Prolab Stuttgart